Sexual offending against children: assessment and treatment of male abusers

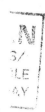

Male sexual offending against children is a serious and widespread problem in Britain and the USA. Increasing awareness of this disturbing fact has led to great public and professional interest in how to deal with sex offenders. *Sexual Offending Against Children: Assessment and Treatment of Male Abusers* is the first book written specifically by UK professionals about practice, and it brings together people experienced in working with sex offenders and their families in a range of community based and institutional settings.

The editors and contributors reflect the development, achievement and challenges of practice in the UK, stressing the multi-disciplinary context in which such practice needs to be undertaken. They describe the assessment, treatment and management of sexual offenders who assault children, and consider the impact of such work on individual practitioners and implications for managers and their agencies. The book covers both the theoretical and practical issues raised by working with those who sexually assault children, and demonstrates clearly the application of research and theory in practice.

With its practical approach, linked to a clear and firm theoretical base, *Sexual Offending Against Children: Assessment and Treatment of Male Abusers* will be invaluable to students, teachers and professionals in Social Work, Social Policy and Psychology, as well as to those in the Police and Prison Services who work with child sexual offenders.

Tony Morrison is an independent social work consultant and trainer, and founder Chair of NOTA, the National Association for the Development of Work with Sex Offenders; **Marcus Erooga** is Manager of the NSPCC Child Protection Team and Child Care Centre in East Lancashire; and **Richard C. Beckett** is a consultant forensic and clinical psychologist and Head of Oxford Forensic Psychology Service.

Sexual offending against children

Assessment and treatment of male abusers

Edited by Tony Morrison, Marcus Erooga
and Richard C. Beckett

Foreword by Valerie Howarth

London and New York

First published 1994
by Routledge
11 New Fetter Lane, London EC4P 4EE

Simultaneously published in the USA and Canada
by Routledge
29 West 35th Street, New York, NY 10001

Reprinted 1995

Typeset in Times by LaserScript, Mitcham, Surrey
Printed and bound in Great Britain by
Mackays of Chatham PLC, Chatham, Kent

British Library Cataloguing in Publication Data
A catalogue record for this book is available from the British Library

Library of Congress Cataloguing in Publication Data
A catalogue record for this book is available from the Library of Congress

ISBN 0–415–05504–0 (hbk)
ISBN 0–415–05505–9 (pbk)

To
Jacquie, Christopher, James and Anna
Caroline
Lucy and Jude

Contents

Illustrations

FIGURES

TABLES

Contributors

Richard Beckett is a consultant forensic and clinical psychologist and Head of Oxford Forensic Psychology service. He has worked as a forensic psychologist for 12 years and has extensive experience in the assessment and treatment of sex offenders, both individually and in groups. In addition to his own group treatment programme he acts as a consultant to a variety of treatment programmes in England involved in the treatment of both adult and adolescent sex offenders.

He has held grants for research into adult and adolescent sex offenders and is co-recipient of Home Office grants into the evaluation of community sex offender treatment programmes in England, and the treatment of sex offenders in English prisons. He sits on the Home Office special advisory panel for the development of sex offender treatment programmes in English prisons and is a member of the research committee of the National Association for the Development of Work with Sex Offenders (NOTA).

David Briggs Ph.D. works for the Special Hospitals Service Authority at Rampton Hospital with responsibility for organisation development.

As a practising clinical psychologist he has run treatment programmes for sexual offenders, both within Rampton and in the community for many years, and has a special interest in the problems of the incarcerated sexual offender with learning difficulties.

Paul Clark is Co-ordinator of the NSPCC in the North West/Lancashire Probation Service 'Partnership Project', working with sex offenders in Lancashire. He was previously a Child Protection Officer in the Oldham NSPCC Child Protection Team, focusing on work with sexually aggressive behaviour.

Between 1985 and 1991 he worked as a Probation Officer in Rochdale and was involved in 1987 in establishing the Rochdale Sex Offenders Groupwork Treatment Programme.

As well as groupwork his experience includes risk assessment, training and consultation to sex offender groupwork programmes. He has also worked with children who have been sexually abused, and their families.

He is currently Chair of the North-West Branch of the National Association for the Development of Work with Sex Offenders (NOTA).

Marcus Erooga is Manager of the NSPCC Child Protection Team and Child Care Centre in East Lancashire. Between 1991 and 1994 he managed the Oldham NSPCC CPT, with a specialist focus developing work with sexually aggressive behaviour against children.

After qualifying with an MA in Social Work in 1983 he worked as a Probation Officer in Greater Manchester before moving to the NSPCC in Rochdale in 1987. Between 1988 and 1993 he was a practitioner in the Rochdale, Oldham and Bury Sex Offenders Groupwork Treatment Programme, and subsequently a member of the programme management committee. He continues to provide case and groupwork programme consultancy as well as training for practitioners and managers. In 1991 he was awarded a Winston Churchill Memorial Trust Travelling Fellowship to study the treatment of sexually aggressive behaviour in North America.

He is an active member of the National Association for the Development of Work with Sex Offenders (NOTA) and between 1992 and 1995 was north-west member of the National Executive Committee.

He has previously published articles about groupwork with sexual offenders, groupwork with mothers of sexually abused children, a booklet on the investigation of physical abuse and neglect, and guidelines for good practice in child protection for probation, published by Greater Manchester Probation Service. He is a member of the Editorial Board of the *Journal of Sexual Aggression.*

Dawn Fisher is a forensic clinical psychologist working with the Regional Forensic Service in the West Midlands. She has worked in the forensic field since 1979, working at Broadmoor Special Hospital for two years prior to qualifying as a clinical psychologist and then with Merseyside Regional Forensic Services.

She has specialised particularly in the assessment and treatment of sex offenders and works with adults and adolescents on an individual and group basis. She is currently involved in a research project for the Home Office to evaluate the effectiveness of community treatment programmes for sex offenders and is developing assessment methods.

She is Vice-Chair of the National Association for the Development of Work with Sex Offenders (NOTA) and convenes the research sub-committee.

Tony Morrison is an independent social work practitioner, trainer and consultant based in Rochdale. Formerly leader of the Rochdale NSPCC team, he has extensive experience of multi-disciplinary child protection work. He has worked with both adult and adolescent sex offenders at the Merseyside Forensic Psychology Service and acts as consultant to several treatment programmes. He was a founder member and first Chair of the National Association for the Development of Work with Sex Offenders (NOTA).

As a consultant he works with managers, both in the UK and overseas, on a range of issues including interagency work, supervision, team building and the management of change. He was a member of the Department of Health Committee on the evaluation of Area Child Protection Committees, and has worked with a number of ACPCs.

His publications include *Supervision in Social Care* (Longman, 1993), and co-authorship of *Dangerous Families* (Tavistock, 1986).

Dave O'Callaghan qualified as a social worker at Lancaster University in 1982 and has worked as a child care practitioner and guardian *ad litem* in the West Midlands and North West. He has been involved in the Greater Manchester Adolescent Programme (G-MAP) since its inception and is currently a Team Manager in Bolton Social Services.

Bobbie Print is a social work consultant who has worked with victims and survivors of child sexual abuse for 12 years. In 1987 she was a member of the multi-disciplinary team that set up the Greater Manchester Adolescent Programme (G-MAP). The programme carries out initial and comprehensive assessments of adolescent sex offenders and offers an offence specific treatment programme to young males who are considered suitable.

In addition to her work with G-MAP, Bobbie has also worked with a number of young people who have sexually abused others. She is a member of the NOTA National Executive Committee.

Gerrilyn Smith is a clinical psychologist and Clinical Director of Limewood Therapeutic Residential Unit for Young Women in London. She was formerly the Course Lecturer for the Department of Health Postgraduate Training Programme in Child Sexual Abuse and held a clinical attachment with the Child Sexual Abuse Team at Great Ormond Street Hospital, London.

Foreword

The most compelling reason for finding ways of successfully treating people who commit sexual offences against children is one of child protection. Programmes to change the behaviour of offenders may have a beneficial effect on the individuals involved and enable them to rejoin society or to be reunited with their families. But for the majority of workers engaged in managing programmes, in improving practice and influencing policy in this difficult area of social concern, the driving motivation is the need of the victims. This is why those who work with child victims and those who treat the perpetrators of child abuse must continually share information and work together.

Since its beginning in 1986, ChildLine has talked with thousands of children and young people about a wide range of problems, and child sexual abuse has always been high in our statistics. ChildLine counsellors have listened to children talking about appalling abuse: betrayed by those who should care for them, made to feel responsible for the actions of the abuser and ashamed of their part in what has happened. Every day our counsellors hear the confusion of children manipulated and used by abusers, children who wish to avoid the break-up of their homes, who suffer the anxiety of being removed and placed into care and most of all who fear that they will not be believed. Most of the agency's work involves intra-familial abuse but we also hear from children caught in the web of the paedophile ring or being forced into dangerous sexual relationships.

Hearing this daily cry of pain from victims, one response might be to call on the legislators and judiciary for longer sentences and retribution. This book is essential reading for those seeking policy solutions; for what we also know from the children is that unless there is an alternative to prison, they often will not tell. Indeed, when abusers serve a prison sentence without treatment they are likely to return to their community and to their abusing behaviour. Imprisonment, where at best the abusers' fantasies are reinforced and, at worst, where further methods of acquiring, grooming and seducing children are learned, does not provide an answer. Those in Parliament and the judiciary will find this book of particular relevance in seeking more appropriate responses, as will senior managers in the community. Where community programmes are set up as an alternative to imprisonment, but the 'therapists' fail to understand the manipulative behaviour of many offenders or are distracted by the emotional impact of the abuser's own abuse, the projects will not only fail but may be dangerous. Planning for a positively managed service demands an understanding of the complex issues involved, issues clearly outlined in *Sexual Offending Against Children: Assessment and Treatment of Male Abusers.*

The Report of the NCH Committee into Children and Young People Who Sexually Abuse Other Children (1992) highlighted the huge resource gap in services for children who have been abused and are abusing. In all its manifestations the issue of child sexual abuse does not appear to be one of serious national concern and yet the indicators show that attention to this problem would reduce a huge amount of pain and misery. Projects treating abusers are often carried out as an additional extra to the workload or are funded by charitable contributions.

During recent years a dedicated group of people has committed itself to finding answers to the treatment problem. Their thinking is reflected in this book which provides a practical guide to the issues, research and current practice in this fast-developing field in the UK. For too long practitioners have had to rely on literature from North America, but here we have a detailed examination of what is possible in this country. In a new and emerging area of practice we are offered an explanation of the causes of sexually abusing behaviour, a theoretical framework within which to understand it and advice on how those working in this personally challenging field of social care should be supported.

If children are to be protected, not only from the abuser but from the often equally disruptive consequences of intervention, then ways of community treatment, albeit separated for some time from the family, must be found for abusers. This is a high-risk option, dependent on sound assessment. It is equally essential that persistent child abusers are identified and that dangerous and disturbed offenders are recognised and treated in security. The following pages provide help in setting a disciplined framework for assessment. If offenders are to be able to return to their families they must receive treatment which confronts the abusing behaviour and which ensures that they take full responsibility, freeing the child from a sense of blame. All of this requires skill, continuous evaluation and personal insight on behalf of the worker. This book outlines much of what is known of good practice, and also demonstrates that if workers in this field are to survive they need care, support and supervision, commodities often lacking in over stretched agencies.

There is still much that we do not know. While the experience of ChildLine confirms the research and intelligence that most abuse is carried out by men, children and young people do call our counsellors to talk of abuse by women and by other children. This book does not detail the work being done in these areas, but it does usefully highlight the need for greater understanding of what is effective in terms of changing behaviour. For example, the work with young male offenders can be based on programmes for adult males, but there is still much we need to know about why young children abuse and the most appropriate way to treat them.

Sexual Offending Against Children: Assessment and Treatment of Male Abusers is a milestone in drawing together many of the key issues relating to the treatment of offenders. It fills a huge gap in UK literature on the subject and should be read by policy makers, practitioners, trainers and children's advocates. The rights of children cannot be met in isolation and only when we are serious about intervention into the addictive and contaminating cycle of abuse will we show ourselves to be serious about protecting the childhood of our young.

Valerie Howarth
Executive Director
ChildLine

Acknowledgements

Many people have contributed, both knowingly and unknowingly, to the creation, evolution and expression of the ideas and practice described in this book. We would, however, like to express some particular thanks and acknowledgements.

First, thank you to all the secretarial staff who patiently typed and retyped drafts, responded to our requests for text to be submitted in particular formats and who fitted this work within their own already busy schedules.

Second, we would like to acknowledge the support and guidance of colleagues who read draft chapters, offered helpful comments, put us back on track and encouraged us to continue.

Third, thank you to family members, both young and old for their encouragement, practical support, patience and tolerance during the long process of bringing the idea of this book to fruition.

Finally, we would like to acknowledge the much wider contribution of colleagues and co-workers throughout this field without whose commitment, skills and sharing of ideas none of us would have been able to progress.

We hope that this book both reflects the extraordinary progress made by them in this field during the last decade, and encourages us all to make further progress in combating sexual offending.

Introduction

Male sexual offending against children is a serious and widespread problem in this country, the vast majority of which still goes unreported. The effects of sexual abuse on children are both enduring and damaging. The causes of offending are complex, resulting from a combination of interpersonal, environmental and societal factors. However, the premise of this book is that males who sexually assault children are responsible for their behaviour and must be held accountable for their actions.

> The time is past when we can count child molesters as harmless fondlers and rapists as innocently misunderstanding the victim's intent, or when we can see the victims as wilfully neglectful or actively seductive. Such excuses for inaction as a society do not withstand even the most casual scrutiny.
>
> (Marshall *et al.*, 1989)

Increasing recognition of the need for action since the mid-1980s has led to a rapid expansion of both professional and public interest in how to deal with sex offenders and has galvanised professional energy into trying to develop effective intervention and treatment of sexually abusive behaviour.

British practitioners and managers have, however, to a great extent remained dependent on North American literature. Valuable though such work is, and will continue to be, it addresses a very different cultural, judicial and service delivery context. The rapid expansion of British practice has made more urgent the need for a text such as this in order to reflect the development, achievement and challenges of practice in the UK. In many ways this book is part of the 'coming of age' of British practice.

The book has primarily been written for practitioners and clinicians from a range of disciplines, as well as for managers wishing to inform themselves about practice and the needs of their staff. It will also be of value to students and teachers involved in professional training and those working with victims of sexual assault who wish to gain a better understanding of sexual abusers.

Based on the extensive experience of the authors it provides a description and analysis of practical approaches to the assessment and treatment of sexual abusers, drawing primarily on a cognitive behavioural approach. The authors would wish to acknowledge that this approach represents a paradigm at this point in the development of our understanding of what is likely to be most effective.

We recognise that sexual assaults against women, and sexual abuse by females and pre-adolescent children, are also serious problems, treatment of which is important. However, the merits of seeking to provide a generalised text which attempts to address all of these issues are outweighed by the need for detailed attention to be given to each of these groups. Readers wishing to consider these issues further are referred to Elliot (1993) and Cunningham and MacFarlane (1991).

Whilst the book has been produced by several authors, it is much more than a collection of edited papers. The structure of the book is progressive, although each chapter will also stand alone to a great extent, so that the reader can choose where to start according to their interest. There are, however, sections where reference is made to material elsewhere in the book with which it is necessary to be familiar in order to fully understand the point being made. Chapter 1, where the key research and theories are discussed, is probably the most essential in this respect. The authorship also reflects the book's commitment to a multi-disciplinary approach and brings together experience in working with sex offenders and their families in a range of community-based and institutional settings.

Given the above, the reader will be aware of different styles in different chapters, which the editors have not sought to eradicate. There are also some issues on which the authors have different opinions. It is hoped this will stimulate readers to consider their own position, in addition to acknowledging that there is not, nor should there be, a homogeneous position presented about the management of such a complex problem. There are some basic issues, however, on which the authorship is agreed, which form the basis of our writing.

Overwhelmingly it is males who abuse their power and role to exploit children for their own sexual and psychological gratification; sexually abusive behaviour is highly self-reinforcing and compulsive in nature; controlling and changing it requires co-ordinated intervention by criminal justice and child protection systems, to ensure that victims are protected, offenders are made accountable for their actions and to create a context for treatment which ensures the protection of the public; the primary and continuing aim of any work with sex offenders is the protection of victims;

and the goal of treatment is not cure, but the development and maintenance of self-control by the offender on a lifelong basis.

Tony Morrison, Marcus Erooga and Richard Beckett

Glossary

In a changing field of work, terminology will continue to develop as ideas and understanding evolve. This glossary is therefore intended to provide consistency in the text, rather than suggesting any definitive use of the terminology.

Client – those in community treatment or non-medical settings.
Contact offences – those where there is physical contact between the offender and victim.
Deviant refers to sexual abuse as defined below.
Extra-familial – offences committed by those outside of the family, including those who have some responsibility for the victim, e.g. babysitters, teachers, etc.
Fixated – those with a sexual and emotional preference for children.
Inmate – those in secure/custodial settings.
Intra-familial – offences against those related by kinship, a member of the same household, or parental relationship (e.g. including cohabitee or stepfather not currently part of the household).
Non-contact offences – those where there is no physical contact between the offender and victim, e.g. indecent exposure.
Non-fixated – those who have no clear preference for sexual contact with children.
Offender/sex offender or **abuser** – anyone who has committed sexual abuse and/or an illegal sexual act involving a child or young person, whether or not this has been reported, or the perpetrator has been cautioned, prosecuted or convicted.
Patient – those in a hospital setting.
Practitioner/therapist/clinician – those having direct contact with offenders in a professional capacity.
Sexual abuse is used to mean actual, or threatened, sexual exploitation of a child or adolescent.

Sexual assault is also used in the above sense, but unless specified is not intended to imply use of force or a physical assault as part of the sexual abuse.

Sexual fantasy – thoughts which generate sexual arousal.

Sexual offending – those behaviours which result in sexual abuse.

Survivor refers to someone who is post-treatment or emotionally/chronologically distant from their sexual abuse. This is usually used to describe adults.

Victim – child or person currently or recently abused. Victims are assumed to be of either gender unless specified.

1 Adult sex offenders

Who are they? Why and how do they do it?

Dawn Fisher

Any consideration of the assessment and treatment of sexual offenders and work with other family members, must be based on an understanding of the available information and models about sexual offending. This chapter, which reviews the current knowledge regarding sex offenders and some of the theories which attempt to explain their behaviour, its development and maintenance, thus provides a basis for the rest of the book. In view of the subject of the book, the primary focus of this chapter is men who sexually assault children, although some reference is made to other groups such as male rapists and women who sexually assault children. Adolescent offenders are considered in Chapter 7.

WHO ARE THEY?

Although the public image of sex offenders tends to oscillate between the extremes of 'dirty old men in raincoats exposing themselves', often regarded as trivial, and 'sadistic child murderers', for whom the public hold the greatest loathing, the vast majority of sex offenders fall in the range between these two extremes and are probably far greater in number than society wishes to acknowledge. However, establishing who they are, how many there are and what exactly they do is fraught with difficulty, as many sex offenders go undetected and those who are detected are frequently characterised by denial and minimisation. Unless provided with assurances of confidentiality, freedom from prosecution or anonymity, offenders themselves are highly unlikely to reveal the true nature and extent of their sexually deviant behaviour. Indeed, those working with sex offenders comment on the problem of the unreliability of self-report (Abel *et al.*, 1981).

What we do know about the facts and figures of sex offending has therefore to be drawn from a number of different sources, primarily incidence and prevalence studies of sexual abuse, official statistics of reported and convicted offences, information from victims and, where available, information from sex offenders themselves.

Prevalence of sexual abuse: official statistics

The problem of under-reporting

Since the response to sexual abuse involves a number of different agencies, primarily the police, probation service, courts, social services, health service departments and voluntary agencies, there is a variety of sources of information available. However, the types of information recorded and the methods of recording used by each agency vary according to their aims and objectives, and are not therefore necessarily comparable. For example, whilst one agency may record each child as a separate case, another will record each family as one case.

The Home Office regularly publishes records of reported offences and convictions, and these are an important source of information about the level of sexual abuse. However, there are a number of problems with their data, so the figures have to be interpreted with caution. The first major difficulty is that these figures only account for reported offences, and in view of the substantial under-reporting of sexual offences, are likely to be an underestimate. Russell (1984) estimated that less than 10 per cent of all sexual assaults are reported to the police and less than 1 per cent result in the arrest, conviction and imprisonment of the offender. She further found that only 2 per cent of incest cases and 6 per cent of extra-familial cases had been reported. The *British Crime Survey* (Home Office, 1988) estimated the report rate for rape and indecent assault as 17 per cent, similar to rates for other crimes against the person. This estimate was arrived at by comparing the results of victim surveys to those of crimes reported to the police and so may again be subject to under-reporting, as victims do not always disclose their abuse. Even when reported, many cases are not prosecuted, due to difficulties in using a child's statement, the victim retracting their statement even though believed, or the offender being cautioned. A further difficulty with the Home Office figures is that they refer to the number of offences, and not the number of offenders. Official figures thus greatly underestimate the incidence of sexual abuse.

Although such statistics are useful in reflecting the patterns and trends of offending, they probably give very misleading information about the types of offences that are being committed. This is because many offenders will only admit to a lesser charge and the difficulties of proving a more serious offence may lead to that charge being dropped. A further problem is that offenders may have committed many offences but are only charged with a few 'specimen' charges.

Whilst reported sex offences increased by 40 per cent between 1979 and 1989, they still only account for less than 1 per cent of recorded crime. In 1989, only 3 per cent of probation orders on males were for sex offences and sex offenders accounted for 8.1 per cent of the male prison population. There were only 23 female sex offenders in prison during that year. Statistics relating to the numbers of sex offenders in prison or on probation are probably most helpful in planning service provision, but provide little help in knowing the extent of the problem in the general population.

Incidence and prevalence of sexual offences against children

Although there are many studies of clinical populations showing high rates of childhood sexual victimisation (Friedman and Harrison, 1984; Coons and Milstein, 1986), it could be argued that such populations represent a biased sample and do not reflect the level of sexual abuse in the general population. Similarly, as discussed above, using the numbers of reported offences can be equally misleading.

Studies which attempt to survey the general population probably provide the truest reflection of the level of sexual abuse. The two methods used to survey this are studies of incidence or prevalence. *Incidence* refers to the number of new cases occurring over a specified time period, usually a year, and based only on reported cases. *Prevalence* refers to retrospective information from subjects about their previous experiences and is also subject to a number of methodological problems. To date there have been very few British studies of either incidence or prevalence, and consequently there has been much reliance on North American research.

Incidence

A study of child sexual abuse in Northern Ireland (Northern Ireland Research Team, 1991) revealed a rate of 0.9 per 1,000. This is comparable to rates from studies in the USA. The American National Incidence Study (NCCAN, 1981) estimated a rate of 0.7 per 1,000, and Sarafino (1979) obtained a rate of 1.2 per 1,000 from four areas of the USA. The Northern Ireland study suggested that a rate of 1.83 per 1,000 children may be a more realistic minimum figure, if suspected cases that had not been proven are taken into account. Given that the study was only based on reported cases, the 'true' incidence rate is almost certainly much higher.

Prevalence

The rates of child sexual abuse revealed by prevalence studies vary enormously, ranging from 7 per cent for both males and females (Fritz *et al.*, 1981) to 62 per cent (Wyatt, 1985). The reasons for the variation are the differing definitions used for sexual abuse, sample characteristics, the interview format and methods of eliciting the information. For example, generally it would appear that studies which employed the use of face-to-face interviews resulted in higher reported rates of sexual abuse. Of particular note in this respect is the study by Russell (1983). Despite using a strict definition of sexual abuse which meant that only 'contact' sexual offences were included, this study found the highest rates. Twenty-eight per cent of females reported having been abused under the age of 14 and 38 per cent under the age of 18, out of a sample of 930 interviewed. In order to make the study comparable to others, Russell added non-contact abuse and the rate rose to 48 per cent for under 14 and 54 per cent for under 18. Studies which included males and females have found a higher rate for females than males. Finkelhor (1979) estimated that 19 per cent of females and 9 per cent of males had been sexually abused before the age of 17. Badgley (1984), in a random survey of the Canadian population, included both males and females. In this study 22 per cent of females and 9 per cent of males reported being abused under the age of 18. Of further note, 20 per cent of females and 9 per cent of males in the survey reported physical injuries during the assault. Badgley concluded that 60 per cent of the victims under 16 had been physically forced or threatened by the offender.

A number of prevalence surveys have now been carried out in Britain. Nash and West (1985), using two samples of females, found that 42 per cent of female patients in a GP practice and 54 per cent of 148 female students reported sexual abuse before the age of 16. In both samples 50 per cent of the abuse involved physical contact.

Baker and Duncan (1985) reported that of their random sample of 2,019 males and females, 12 per cent of the females and 8 per cent of the males had been sexually abused before the age of 16. Kelly (1991) surveyed 1,244 British college students using a questionnaire. They reported that before the age of 18, 59 per cent of females and 27 per cent of males had experienced at least one unwanted sexual incident. When exhibitionism, abuse attempts which were successfully resisted and 'less serious' forms of abuse by peers were excluded, the prevalence figures were 21 per cent for females and 7 per cent for males. Despite the variations in the different studies, all reveal that sexual abuse is a serious problem, affecting a significant proportion of the population.

Potential levels of abusers in the population

The high percentages of the general population who report having been sexually abused, together with the fact that only a tiny proportion are reported to the authorities and an even smaller number convicted, suggest that the number of sex offenders in the population is significant. One way to estimate the percentage of the population who could be potential sex offenders comes from studies that focus on 'normal' samples (non-sex offenders) and investigate those characteristics e.g. sexual attitudes, which they share with known sexual offenders. The majority of these studies have used college students. However, as the majority of students tend to have come from middle-class socio-economic groups, they cannot be regarded as representative of the general population. Briere and Runtz (1989) suggest that studies using students might be a 'conservative test of hypotheses' regarding motivation for sexual abuse, as they probably represent a less deviant sample than incarcerated sex offenders. It is also possible that they represent a less deviant sample than the population as a whole. A number of studies have investigated the percentage of college males who self-report that they would commit an act of forced sexual aggression if they could ensure that they would not be caught or punished. Malamuth (1981) estimated that 35 per cent of college males reported the likelihood of rape if assured of not being caught or punished. Subjects in Petty and Dawson's study (1989) also reported it unlikely that they would be caught and punished if they did carry out a rape.

Rapaport and Burkhart (1984) found that 28 per cent of college males had engaged in sexually coercive activity. Muehlenard and Linton (1987) reported that over 77 per cent of college females had been involved as victims and 50 per cent of college males as perpetrators of sexually abusive acts.

Regarding attitudes towards the acceptability of rape, Goodchilds and Zellman (1984) found in their study that the majority of males in their high school sample reported that 'date rape' was acceptable under a variety of circumstances.

Further studies have demonstrated that deviant sexual arousal profiles may be obtained from non-sex offenders under certain circumstances, particularly when angry (Yates *et al.*, 1984), under the influence of alcohol (Barbaree *et al.*, 1983) or given permissive instructions (Quinsey *et al.*, 1981).

Regarding the arousal to, or abuse of children, Briere and Runtz (1989) found that 21 per cent of college males reported having some sexual attraction to children and 7 per cent reported some likelihood of having sex with a child if they could ensure not being detected or punished. Finkelhor and Lewis (1988) estimated that 10 per cent of males from the sample of their telephone survey had admitted having sexually abused a child. Fromuth *et al.* (1991) surveyed 582 college males, 3 per cent of whom reported having abused a child.

These studies clearly demonstrate that a significant percentage of the 'normal' male population believe it acceptable to carry out a sexual assault, and report the likelihood of doing so if they could be assured of not being detected or punished. A percentage also report having actually carried out forced sexual assaults against both women and children. Given that the samples used tended to be male college students, and the likelihood that subjects would be prone to under-report, the base rate in the general population is likely to be significantly higher.

What sex offenders tell us about themselves

Although sex offenders' self-reporting is fraught with difficulty due to their denial and minimisation, some very important studies, which have been able to offer assurances of confidentiality and immunity from prosecution, have uncovered a wealth of information which probably reflects a more accurate picture of the nature and extent of sex offenders' behaviours.

Kaplan (1985) demonstrated the importance in research of offering confidentiality to sex offenders. The same subjects, offenders on parole, were interviewed in two settings. The first interview, in the criminal justice setting, revealed only 5 per cent of the sex offences that the subjects later admitted in the mental health setting where confidentiality was offered. In addition to reporting many more offences, subjects also admitted a greater variety of sex offences. Abel *et al.* (1983) reported that their subjects admitted 20 per cent more types of sexual deviancy when reinterviewed by experienced interviewers, thus demonstrating the effect of interviewers on results. Abel *et al.* (1987) also found much higher rates of sex offending in their study of 561 non-incarcerated sex offenders, the most comprehensive self-report study to date. They employed elaborate measures to offer a high level of confidentiality. Given that only a small number of offenders are detected, and only a small number of these are imprisoned, it was considered important to use non-incarcerated offenders as a more representative sample. Incarcerated offenders were also thought less likely to be truthful, for fear of adversely affecting their chances of parole if they revealed further offending. This study represented a watershed in the knowledge base about sex offenders, because of the huge amount of previously unknown information revealed, and served to dispel some previously held ideas and stereotypes. This one study has probably affected professional attitudes and decision making in regard to sex offenders more profoundly than any other, and will therefore be reviewed in some detail. Some important features will also be discussed in comparison with other research.

Demographic variables

The subjects in the study ranged in age from 13 to 76 years, with an average age of 31.5 years. The majority were moderately educated, with 40 per cent having completed one year of college. Half of the subjects had formed a significant relationship with an adult partner, leading to marriage or an ongoing 'living with' relationship. Sixty-five per cent were fully employed, and only 11 per cent had been unemployed for more than one month. The subjects were representative of the ethnic subgroups of the general population and came from all socio-economic levels.

It is a general finding of surveys of sex offender populations that variables such as level of intelligence, age, ethnicity, education and psychiatric status do not differ significantly from the rates in the general populations from which the samples are drawn (Wolf, 1984).

Regarding ethnicity, very little has been written about the representation of ethnic groups in sex offenders as a whole. However, it has been noted that there is an over-representation of black and other ethnic minorities in rapist populations (Dietz, 1978; Vinogradov *et al.*, 1988). It has been suggested that this over-representation is due to ethnic groups being subject to more scrutiny and treated more harshly by the authorities (Grubin and Gunn, 1990).

A consistent finding across studies is the unusually high number of convicted child abusers who were themselves abused sexually as children, compared to the number in the non-sex offending population. In 1984 Abel *et al.* reported that 24 per cent of the child abusers who assaulted females and 40 per cent who assaulted males had a history of sex victimisation. Whilst there is some variation in the rates of sexual abuse found across a range of studies, the rates tend to be below 50 per cent, which also demonstrates that a substantial number of child abusers have not been sexually abused.

Extent of offending

The 561 sex offenders in Abel *et al.*'s (1987) study self-reported an astonishing number of offences. Table 1.1 shows the number of completed paraphilic acts and victims for different categories of paraphilia. A paraphilia is

characterised by arousal in response to sexual objects or situations that are not part of normative arousal activity patterns and whose essential features are intense sexual urges and sexually arousing fantasies generally involving non-human objects, the suffering or humiliation of one's self or one's partner, or children or other non-consenting persons.

(American Psychiatric Association, 1987)

It is important to note that although this study revealed a huge amount of offending, the majority of individuals offended against a few victims on few occasions, and it was a minority who accounted for huge numbers of victims and offences. It can also be seen that the number of paraphilic acts and the number of victims is related to the type of paraphilia. For example, non-incest offenders targeting boys committed the greatest number of crimes but offended against each victim less frequently than incest offenders targeting females, who had fewer victims but offended against each victim many times.

Table 1.1 Completed paraphilic acts and victims/partners by diagnosis

Paraphilia	Number of subjects seen	Total completed paraphilic acts	% of total completed paraphilic acts	Total victims	% of total victims
1 Paedophilia (non-incest) female target	224	5,197	1.8	4,435	2.3
2 Paedophilia (non-incest) male target	153	43,100	14.8	22,981	11.8
3 Paedophilia (incest) female target	159	12,927	4.4	286	0.2
4 Paedophilia (incest) male target	44	2,741	0.9	75	0.0
5 Rape	126	907	0.3	882	0.5
6 Exhibitionism	142	71,696	24.6	72,974	37.3
7 Voyeurism	62	29,090	10.0	26,648	13.6
8 Frottage	62	52,669	18.1	55,887	28.6
9 Obscene mail	3	3	0.0	3	0.0
10 Transsexualism	29	5,539	1.9	12	0.0
11 Transvestitism	31	20,779	7.1	NA	NA
12 Fetishism	19	6,863	2.4	160	0.1
13 Sadism	28	3,800	1.3	132	0.1
14 Masochism	17	19,366	6.6	37	0.0
15 Homosexuality [sic]	24	3,701	1.3	2	0.0
16 Obscene phone calling	19	2,578	0.9	1,955	1.0
17 Public masturbation	17	6,423	2.2	6,870	3.5
18 Bestiality	14	3,114	1.1	1,676	0.9
19 Urolagnia	4	409	0.1	385	0.2
20 Coprophilia	4	107	0.0	7	0.0
21 Arousal to odours	2	728	0.3	NA	NA
Total		291,737	100.1	195,407	100.1

Source: Abel *et al.* (1987). Reprinted with permission.

Multiple offence categories and age of onset

Table 1.2 shows the percentage of paraphiliacs with multiple paraphilias. This highlights the high level of cross-over between different sexually deviant behaviours. Previously it had been largely assumed that sex offenders only indulged in one type of deviant behaviour and had specific preferences for victims. This study revealed that 23.3 per cent of the subjects offended against both family and non-family victims. Twenty per cent of the subjects offended against both sexes and 26 per cent used both touching and non-touching behaviours when offending. This finding highlights the importance of conducting a thorough assessment in order to investigate the possibility of a wider range of offending.

A further finding of this study which has caused much controversy is the age of onset of deviant sexual interests. In Abel's study 53.6 per cent of subjects reported the onset of at least one deviant sexual interest prior to age 18. Furthermore each subject reported two paraphilias by the time he reached adulthood. This is reinforced by increasing evidence of the number of offences committed by adolescents, as discussed in Chapter 7.

In contrast to Abel *et al.*, Marshall and Eccles (1991) report that in their sample of 129 outpatient child abusers, only 29 per cent reported having deviant fantasies prior to age 20. They also found a much smaller number of multiple paraphilias. However, when Marshall and Eccles reclassified their sample and selected those subjects who admitted to having abused at least four victims, they found that 80 per cent of those offenders had committed their first offence prior to age 20, and 36 per cent had multiple paraphilias. As a group, however, Marshall's sample were much less deviant than that studied by Abel *et al.* As discussed previously, it may also be that the elaborate confidentiality assurances offered by the Abel study contributed to the much higher rates of disclosure of the nature and extent of deviant behaviours.

Weinrott and Saylor (1991) used a computer-administered interview to explore the past criminal behaviour of 99 institutionalised sex offenders. As with other self-report studies, many more undetected sexual offences were disclosed, consistent with Abel's study. In addition they also explored the incidence of prior non-sexual offending and found a high rate of non-sexual offences committed by the sample of men in the year prior to conviction. To some extent the anti-social nature of rapists was anticipated, but the researchers were surprised by the high level of criminality present in the child abusers, particularly those whose only known crime was incest.

Table 1.2 Percentage of paraphiliacs with multiple paraphilias

Diagnosis	N	Number of paraphilias									
		1	2	3	4	5	6	7	8	9	10
Paedophilia (non-incest) female target	224	15.2	23.7	19.2	14.7	9.4	4.5	6.7	3.1	1.3	2.2
Paedophilia (non-incest) male target	153	19.0	26.8	19.6	12.4	4.6	3.9	6.5	3.9	0.7	2.6
Paedophilia (incest) female target	159	28.3	25.8	17.0	5.7	8.2	3.8	5.0	1.9	0.6	3.8
Paedophilia (incest) male target	44	4.5	15.9	20.5	18.2	13.6	6.8	9.1	2.3	0.0	9.1
Rape	126	27.0	17.5	19.0	12.7	7.1	3.2	7.9	1.6	1.6	2.4
Exhibitionism	142	7.0	20.4	22.5	15.5	7.0	7.0	9.2	4.9	2.8	3.5
Voyeurism	62	1.6	9.7	27.4	14.5	12.9	8.1	11.3	8.1	3.2	3.2
Frottage	62	21.0	16.1	12.9	16.1	11.3	3.2	12.9	3.2	0.0	3.2
Transsexualism	29	51.7	31.0	13.8	3.4	0.0	0.0	0.0	0.0	0.0	0.0
Transvestitism	31	6.5	29.0	29.0	9.7	0.0	6.5	12.9	0.0	6.5	0.0
Fetishism	19	0.0	15.8	21.1	15.8	26.3	5.3	10.5	0.0	5.3	0.0
Sadism	28	0.0	17.9	28.6	14.3	14.3	3.6	3.6	3.6	7.1	7.1
Masochism	17	0.0	41.2	11.8	5.9	11.8	5.9	5.9	5.9	5.9	5.9
Homosexuality	24	25.0	41.7	25.0	4.2	0.0	0.0	0.0	4.2	0.0	0.0
Obscene phone calling	19	5.3	5.3	21.1	21.1	5.3	10.5	15.8	5.3	5.3	5.3
Public masturbation	17	5.9	17.6	0.0	17.6	17.6	17.6	5.9	5.9	5.9	5.9

Source: Abel et al. (1988), 'Multiple paraphilic diagnoses among sex offenders', Bulletin of the American Academy of Psychiatry and the Law, 16: 153–68. Reprinted after revision with permission.

Female sex offenders

It is widely believed that the vast majority of sexual abuse is perpetrated by males and that female sex offenders only account for a tiny proportion of offences. Indeed, with 3,000 adult male sex offenders in prison in England and Wales at any one time, the corresponding figure for female sex offenders is 12! As such, they have attracted little attention and very little has been written about them.

Finkelhor and Russell (1984) attempted to obtain an incidence figure of female sexual abuse by re-examining the figures from two incidence studies, the American Humane Association (AHA, 1978) and the National Incidence Study (NCCAN, 1981). Due to differing definitions, comparison of the figures is problematic and when the data were re-analysed to omit cases where females 'allowed', as opposed to committed, the abuse, the percentages dropped significantly. The AHA study (op. cit.) reported that 6 per cent of female victims and 14 per cent of male victims were abused by a female acting alone.

Russell (1984) found a higher proportion of female adolescents committing single offences than males, as did Faller (1990), who also estimated that between 5 and 15 per cent of abuse is perpetrated by females generally. Kelly et al. (1991) found much higher rates of abuse by females in their study of British college students. Fifteen per cent of the abuse by peers and 5 per cent of the abuse by adults was perpetrated by females. It was notable that the majority of the victims were male, with only two females reporting such abuse. Of further note is the fact that 62 per cent of the males who reported abuse by a female stated that they were not at all, or only a little, traumatised by the experience. Russell (1984) has suggested that abuse by females may be less traumatic than abuse by males, as they use less force, abuse less often and tend to be closer in age to their victims. However, as Fromuth and Burkhart (1987) suggest, it may also be that males are less likely to define themselves as victimised when abused by females, and a number may construe the experience as positive. This may be due to the effect of cultural pressure on males to regard any heterosexual activity as positive.

Regarding the nature of sexual offending by women, all of the available studies are of very small samples. Barnett *et al.* (1989) found all six of the women in their treatment group had offended with male accomplices, whilst Mathews *et al.* (1989) found only 50 per cent to have done so, in a sample of 16 women. McCarthy (1981) reported that all seven cases in his sample involved at least one male accomplice. Whilst it would be unwise to generalise from such small samples, they do emphasise the importance of devoting further research and clinical resources to improve knowledge and practice in this area. In the final analysis, however, it is unlikely that female sex offenders will be found to account for anything like the amount of offending as male offenders.

Recidivism of male offenders

Limits of current research

The issue of recidivism is of crucial importance to all those involved in work with sex offenders. For those involved in treating sex offenders, the basic test of treatment efficacy is to compare reoffence rates of treated sex offenders against those of untreated sex offenders. For those involved in decision making about the most effective management of sex offenders, knowledge of recidivism rates and those factors which contribute to it is essential. Unfortunately, due to the problems of obtaining an accurate picture, discussed above, this is an area where the results of research have been both varied and controversial.

One of the problems of reviewing studies of recidivism is that the exact nature of the population being studied may not be precisely defined. As different categories of untreated offenders have different reoffence rates (incest offenders 4–10 per cent, rapists 7–35 per cent, non-familial child abusers 10–29 per cent against females and 13–40 per cent against boys, exhibitionists 41–71 per cent (Marshall and Barbaree, 1990a)), the results of such studies may be highly misleading. Some studies of treated offenders can also be criticised because they may only be based on a highly pre-selected group, who may have a low recidivism rate anyway, and often exclude those offenders who did not successfully complete treatment. Further problems concern the fact that control groups are often unavailable and the methods by which recidivism is calculated vary according to whether official or unofficial records are used.

Length of follow-up is another important factor, as typically longer follow-ups give higher recidivism rates. Soothill and Gibbons (1978) found that in a sample of 174 untreated sex offenders followed up over a period of 23 years, the sexual recidivism rate of 11 per cent for 0–5 years rose dramatically to 22 per cent for 5–22 years. Similarly, Marshall and Barbaree (1990a) reported that at two years, the recidivism rate for child abusers was 5.5 per cent for those treated and 12.5 per cent for those untreated, whilst at four years or more the rate had increased to 25 per cent for treated and 64.3 per cent for untreated. Marshall and Barbaree suggest that follow-ups of less than two years are inadequate.

Intra-familial offenders appear to show the lowest levels of recidivism compared to other categories of sex offenders, with rates varying from 4 to

`10 per cent. However, it may be that the follow-up period was not long enough to pick up abuse of the next generation in the family.

Influence of prior conviction on recidivism

Although some of these studies have attempted to select specific populations of sex offenders for study, there remains the problem of them including subjects with a range of criminal histories. Phillpots and Lancucki (1979) report that, using a six-year follow-up of 2,391 untreated English men convicted for the first time for a sexual offence, the reconviction rate was only 1.5 per cent. In contrast, for men who had one previous conviction for a sexual offence, the rate rose to 10.3 per cent and for those with two or more previous sexual convictions the reconviction rate was 22.3 per cent.

Looking at the influence of previous convictions on recidivism, Thornton and Travers (1991) reported on a longitudinal study of recidivism in convicted, but presumably untreated sex offenders. They used a sample of adult male sex offenders discharged from prisons in England and Wales in 1980 from a sentence of at least four years imposed in relation to a sexual offence. This study revealed different patterns of reoffending which clearly showed that violence and previous convictions were closely associated with sexual recidivism.

Recidivism in treated sexual offenders

Marshall and Barbaree (1990a) have examined recidivism in treated offenders and have taken account of such factors as previous offence history, type of offence, length of follow-up and method of follow-up. Studying four outpatient programmes in detail they compared the recidivism rates for rapists, exhibitionists and non-familial child abusers, differentiating when they could between abusers of boys and girls. (See Table 1.3.)

In considering the recidivism rates for the different treatment programmes, it should be borne in mind that the populations in the programmes varied according to different selection criteria. Thus offenders seen as being at high risk of reoffending within the community were excluded from Wolf's and Maletzky's programmes, and because all the programmes required payment for treatment, there was a bias towards white, middle-class offenders. Abel *et al.*'s (1988b) sample appeared far more deviant, and therefore high-risk, compared with the other programmes and was notable in that the drop-out rate was very high (35 per cent).

In order to obtain a more accurate estimate of recidivism, Marshall and

Table 1.3 Recidivism data for outpatient programmes

Programmes	Group†	Per cent reoffending		Data source	Length of follow-up		
		Treated	Untreated		Range	Mean	
1. Northwest Treatment Clinic Wolf (1984)	CMg (N=67)	4.5	—	Probation reports	1–28 months	13.5 months	
	CMb (N=17)	0	—				
	Rapists (N=3)	0	—				
	Exhibitionists (N=27)	14.8	—				
2. Portland Sexual Abuse Clinic Maletzky (1987)	CMg (N=1719)	5.3	—	Official police records	1–14 years	Mode =3+ years	
	CMb (N=513)	13.6	—				
	Rapists (N=87)	26.5	—				
	Exhibitionists (N=462)	6.9	—				
3. Abel's Clinic Abel et al. (1988b)	CMg,b (N=98)	12.2	—	Patient's self-reports	1 year	1 year	
4. Kingston Sexual Behaviour Clinic Marshall and Barbaree (1988)	CMg (N=49)	17.9	42.9	Offical police records plus unofficial records of police and child protection agencies	12–117 months	48 months	
	CMb (N=29)	13.3	42.9		12–109 months	49 months	
	Incest (N=48)	8.0	21.7		12–93 months	34 months	
	Exhibitionists (N=44)	47.8	66.7		14–125 months	57 months	

† CMg, men who molest non-familial girls; CMb, men who molest non-familial boys

Barbaree therefore gathered data from a variety of sources; self-report of the offender, official charge records from the police and reports of suspected reoffences from the unofficial files of both the police and child protection agencies. The recidivism rate determined by combining official charges and unofficial files was 2.4 times greater for child abusers and 2.8 times greater for exhibitionists than the rates from the official records alone. Thus, Marshall and Barbaree argue, this factor should be applied to the other programmes in order to make meaningful comparisons. The results (shown in Table 1.3) also indicate that some programmes seem more successful with one type of client group than others. This finding has a number of implications, not least that practitioners need to be aware that not all offenders will necessarily benefit from the treatment programme they offer. Sex offenders, even those who offend against children, are not a homogeneous group and consequently have a variety of treatment needs which may not be addressed by all treatment programmes. However, it does give rise to a degree of optimism that treatment, if properly planned, targeted and delivered, can be effective in reducing recidivism.

Predictive factors

Regarding factors predictive of recidivism, Abel *et al.* (1988b) found that five factors correctly predicted outcome in 85.7 per cent of their sample, although the limited follow-up period of one year must be borne in mind. The most powerful factor which correctly classified 83.7 per cent of the sample was that of assaulting both boys and girls. The other important factors were failing to accept increased communication with adults as a goal of therapy; committing both contact and non-contact behaviours; being divorced and assaulting both familial and non-familial victims. Barbaree and Marshall (1988) analysed similar data to Abel *et al.* (1988b) and found that socio-economic class, age of victims, educational level, intellectual level and, surprisingly, number of previous offences did not predict recidivism. However, in untreated offenders there was more likelihood of recidivism in offenders of low intellect. Barbaree and Marshall found only two factors which predicted recidivism in treated offenders. Being over the age of 40 was a powerful predictor of non-reoffending in non-familial offenders, but not incest offenders. If the offender had genital-to-genital/anal contact with victims and had assaulted female children, then reoffending after discharge from treatment was more likely than for other sexual offenders. As can be seen from the above studies, recidivism is a complex subject and rates vary according to a number of factors. It is essential in making claims about the likelihood of future offending by either treated or untreated offenders that all of these factors are taken into consideration, to avoid misleading information being used which could have serious ramifications in the management of sex offenders.

WHY AND HOW DO THEY DO IT? THEORIES OF SEXUAL OFFENDING

The one question that is probably asked about sex offenders more than any other is 'Why do they do it?'. Much time and effort has gone into developing theories to explain sex offending behaviour, in the hope that understanding what led to the behaviour will inform treatment. Although a number of treatment techniques have been developed which appear effective with certain types of sex offenders (Marshall, Ward *et al.*, 1991), theories to explain the behaviour are far less satisfactory. However, in treating the problem of sexual offending the question of how the individual came to offend becomes the key issue. This section will examine both of these issues. One of the difficulties in developing an explanation of sexual offending is that many of the theories offered do not adequately define the behaviour they are 'explaining'. Given the diverse range of sexual offending behaviours and the fact that a number of offenders commit a range of different sexual offences, there is a confusion as to whether there should be one theory to explain all offenders, or a theory to explain each type of behaviour. It is therefore not surprising that single-factor theories – biological (Goodman, 1987), psychodynamic (Freud, 1948), sociological (Herman, 1981) or behavioural (Laws and Marshall, 1990) – are seen as inadequate to account for all types of sexual offenders.

Multi-factorial models

The limitations of single-factor theories have resulted in several multi-factorial models being proposed which, whilst not perfect, have proved more helpful in understanding the development of deviant sexual behaviour. These incorporate a number of causal factors, each of which may contribute to the development of deviant sexual behaviour. It is suggested that the key models which are critically reviewed here are also read in the original, where they are set out in full. Unless otherwise stated, the models are applicable to both adult and adolescent offenders.

A good example of how different factors may interact to lead to sexual aggression is provided by Marshall and Barbaree (1990a) who proposed an integrated theory of the aetiology of sexual offending in males which brings together biological, sociological, cultural and situational factors. They suggest that males are conferred biologically with a capacity to sexually aggress which must be overcome by appropriate training to instil social inhibitions toward such behaviour. Variations in hormonal functioning may make this task more or less difficult. Poor parenting, particularly the use of inconsistent and harsh discipline in the absence of love typically fails to instil these constraints and may even serve to facilitate the fusion of sex and aggression rather than separate these two tendencies.

Marshall and Barbaree propose that socio-cultural attitudes may then interact with inadequate socialisation to increase the likelihood of offending and that situational factors can lead to offending.

The criticisms of this model are that it only addresses aggressive sexual behaviour, thus assuming that all forms of sexual offending are expressions of aggression, and it offers no explanation of sexual offending in females. With those exceptions, however, it provides a very plausible and coherent account.

Two models which have become very popular with UK practitioners are those of Wolf (1984) and Finkelhor (1984). Their popularity is probably associated with the fact that they both attempt to explain not only the development of the behaviour, but the process whereby the offence takes place. Although they are separate models they are complementary to each other in many ways and tend to be used as such in the UK.

The basic premise of Wolf's model, which draws together social, developmental, situational and cultural factors, is that early history leads to the development of a particular type of personality which predisposes the individual to developing deviant sexual interests. Wolf suggests that sexual offenders have a history of early experiences of victimisation, either physical or emotional abuse, sexualisation and neglect, and grew up in dysfunctional families. He proposes that it is exposure to the attitudes of abuse of any sort that is important, rather than personal experience of abuse. He suggests that these early experiences of abuse act as 'potentiators' to developing deviant sexual behaviour, as they result in the child learning inappropriate ways of behaving, as well as developing a self-image and belief system where adult males, having power, can do as they want. These potentiators all lessen inhibitions against deviant sexual behaviour such as fear of discovery, harm to victims or social taboos, and the more potentiators are present, the higher the risk of becoming a sexual offender in adult life.

The potentiators lead to a certain type of personality development which Wolf sees as characteristic of sexual offenders in general. Typically this includes egocentricity, a poor self-image, defensiveness, distorted thinking, being ruminative to the point of becoming obsessive in thoughts and behaviour, socially alienated and sexually preoccupied. The individual constantly compares his ideal self with his own poor self-image and as a result views himself as being unable to cope and as failing in many situations. The offender has a tendency to blame external factors for things which go wrong and has a strong need for tightly structured social situations in which he can exercise control and thus lessen anxiety.

Wolf proposes that sexual offenders are also prone to sexualise the behaviour of others. They have learned that sex can act as a form of escapism, with sexual fantasy blocking out other uncomfortable feelings, such as those associated with not coping with situations. Due to their previous experiences in childhood, they will therefore fantasise about deviant sexual behaviour and masturbate when feeling vulnerable. As a result, levels of inhibition against deviant sexual behaviour are decreased, while the level of attraction for the behaviour is increased. Other disinhibitors such as alcohol, drugs or pornography may be used in similar ways by the offender to enhance arousal, also increasing the likelihood of acting on the fantasy.

In order to explain the relationships between all these factors the concept of a 'sexual assault cycle' has been developed, as it was recognised that whilst not all offenders' behaviour was the same, there were common patterns of behaviour. This cycle was originally adapted by Lane and Zamora (1978) from a general cognitive-behavioural dysfunction cycle for specific use with adolescent sex offenders. It has since become a very popular framework for practitioners to use with both adult and adolescent sex offenders, to explore the link between their distorted thinking, compensatory feelings and abusive behaviours, and thus to gain a better understanding of the process by which the offence was committed. Wolf (1984) also formulated a model of a sexual assault 'cycle' based on his experience of work with adult offenders, represented in Figure 1.1.

Wolf's cycle of offending

Typically the cycle begins with the offender having a very negative self-image, such that when a situation arises which he has difficulty coping with, he uses inappropriate coping strategies based on distorted thinking about the problem. Due to this poor self-image he expects to fail or be rejected, and to defend against this he isolates himself. To cope with the isolation the offender indulges in escapist sexual fantasies in order to feel better and provide an illusion that he is in control. These fantasies involve deviant sexual activities and at some point are likely to be reinforced by masturbation. There may also be associated distorted thinking in order to alleviate guilt experienced as a result of indulging in deviant fantasies.

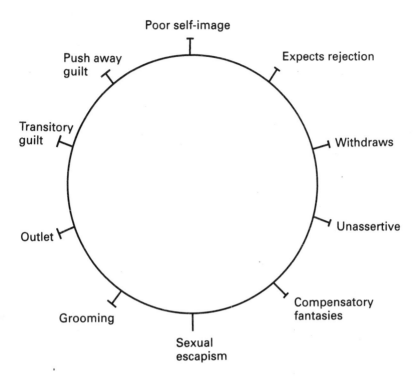

Figure 1.1 Wolf's cycle of offending

Such distorted thoughts are a feature of sex offenders' thinking and occur throughout the cycle.

The offender then progresses to planning the offence and setting up a situation in which abuse can take place. Offenders may go to elaborate lengths to select and prepare, or 'groom' potential victims, and find or create situations where there is least risk of detection. The abuse itself is characterised by a focus on their own needs and wishes, and may increase in severity, or intrusiveness, over time. Once they have committed the offence, itself a highly reinforcing event, the diminished sexual excitement following ejaculation (either as part of the abuse or subsequently through masturbation), is followed by a period of transitory guilt as the offender becomes increasingly aware of the reality of his situation. In seeking to reconstitute his self-image the offender typically uses further distorted thinking to alleviate the guilt and anxiety, by minimising or justifying the abuse and promising himself that he will not do the same again. However, underlying this he is left with the knowledge that he has committed a sexual offence, resulting in further damage to his self-esteem, bringing him back to the feelings he had at the start of the cycle.

Wolf regards an understanding of an individual's cycle as a crucial part of assessment and treatment. Offenders who progress round the cycle quickly i.e. taking hours or days, as opposed to months or years, or whose fantasies become more serious over time, are viewed as presenting a higher risk of reoffending. Due to the repetitive and reinforcing nature of elements of the cycle, sexual offending may be seen as being similar to other forms of addictive behaviours such as alcoholism or compulsive gambling. Wolf regards sexual offending as addictive, in terms of it being compulsive as opposed to leading to pharmacological dependence, and in no way sees this as an excuse for the behaviour.

Although this model appears to be widely applicable, there remain a number of offenders whose developmental history and offending behaviour it does not fit. It also does not adequately explain why victims of physical abuse should develop deviant sexual fantasies rather than purely violent fantasies. It is further limited by not taking account of the fact that many males with a history of victimisation (see earlier discussion) do not go on to become sexual offenders and so offers no explanation of how they differ from those who do. Finally, although very useful for the majority of sex offenders, the sexual assault cycle could be said to provide too rigid a format to cover all sex offenders. However, Wolf's model has proved extremely influential and helpful to many practitioners and offenders in treatment, as it goes a long way to providing a framework within which to understand and intervene in an individual's sexual offending.

Finkelhor's four-factor framework and four preconditions

The other prominent model in the UK is that developed by David Finkelhor (1984). He also proposes a framework, both of factors to explain why adults become sexually interested in children and a model of the process by which an offence is committed. The four-factor framework and the model are often regarded as a single model, but in the original are described separately, and so will be considered here in the same way. Because in the four-factor framework Finkelhor views the factors as complementary rather than as competing explanations, he suggests that they can account for the diversity of the behaviour and backgrounds of offenders.

Factor 1 concerns the emotional congruence that child abusers appear to have with children. There is considerable evidence that children have a special meaning for child abusers, in that they represent weak and non-threatening objects (Howells, 1979). Overcoming the offender's own

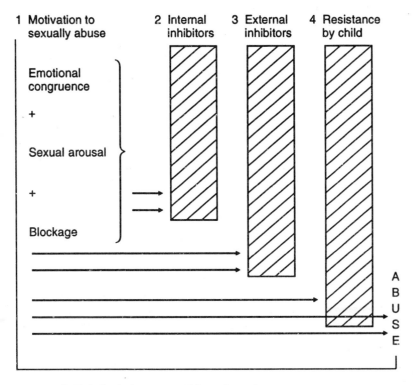

Figure 1.2 Finkelhor's four preconditions of sex abuse

childhood trauma through repetition and identification with the aggressor are also cited as being important factors leading to emotional congruence to children, as evidenced by those offenders who have a history of abuse in their background.

Factor 2 describes the processes whereby an adult would come to find a child sexually arousing. There is much evidence that compared to a 'normal' population, many extra-familial child molesters find children more sexually arousing than adults, as measured by physiological testing. The results with intra-familial offenders have, however, not been consistent, with Abel *et al.* (1981) finding arousal to children and Marshall *et al.* (1986) finding lower arousal to adults, rather than increased arousal to children. The fact that many offenders have a history of sexual abuse is often cited as evidence that attraction to deviant stimuli has been conditioned or modelled through such early childhood sexual experiences. However, it does not explain those who have not been subject to childhood sexual abuse who do sexually offend.

Factor 3 addresses the question of why some offenders are blocked in their ability to meet their sexual and emotional needs in appropriate consenting adult relationships. Two sorts of blockage are described. First, developmental blockage occurs where offenders cannot relate appropriately to peers. There is evidence (Panton, 1978) that child abusers have problems relating to adult females and some studies indicate poor social skills and sexual anxieties being particularly significant for offenders against females. Second, situational blockage occurs where an appropriate relationship exists but for some reason there cannot be any sexual activity with the appropriate partner. However, it would be a gross oversimplification to suggest that blockage in an adult relationship would lead to abuse of children without a pre-existing sexual interest and would be an invitation to offenders to excuse their behaviour or blame their adult partners.

Factor 4 considers the explanations as to why the normal inhibitions against having sexual contact with a child are either overcome or not present in sexual offenders. Lack of impulse control has been suggested to be important, but has only been found in a small number of offenders. Also, given the fact that many offenders admit to detailed planning of offences it is unlikely to be a major factor. Senility and learning difficulties have also been regarded as possible disinhibitors, but again the evidence from research does not bear this out, as only a small number of offenders have such difficulties.

There is much evidence that alcohol plays a disinhibiting role in the commission of many sexual offences, either by having a physiological disinhibiting effect or by having some social meaning which allows the offender to disregard the taboos against the behaviour. However, it is argued that although alcohol may act as a disinhibitor, it does not explain the motivation to abuse which is a prerequisite to sexual offending.

The other explanation which has some empirical support is that of the 'incest avoidance mechanism'. It is hypothesised that stepfathers are less inhibited from having sexual feelings towards a child than natural fathers, either because of different norms or different exposure to the child at an early age. The incidence of abuse by stepfathers is certainly far higher than that for natural fathers.

The question of why someone becomes a sexual offender is complex, resulting from a number of factors operating at different levels. Finkelhor regards the four-factor model as a framework in which to organise the various theories explaining child sexual abuse. The major shortcoming of Finkelhor's framework is that it does not consider the issue of female offenders. However, it does bring together a body of knowledge concerning sexual offenders and attempts to explain how deviant sexual interests arise. As such it makes a major contribution to our theoretical understanding of this issue.

Finkelhor has developed a further four-stage model to describe the necessary preconditions for an offence to occur. In some ways this is akin to the sexual assault cycle, and is often used in conjunction with it in the UK.

1 **Motivation to abuse sexually** In order for any sexual offence to occur, the offender must be motivated to carry out such an act. The motivation is seen as arising from a number of sources, which vary according to the individual's experiences and situation which are variously described in the four-factor framework. This is very similar to Wolf's description of the development of deviant sexual arousal which leads to beginning the assault cycle. The aims of treatment in relation to altering motivation would be to modify the offender's deviant arousal so that they are no longer motivated to offend, as discussed in Chapter 4.

2 **Overcoming internal inhibitions** There are a number of individuals who find deviant sexual activity arousing but who do not offend, presumably because of their internal inhibitions, such as those who report that they would if they could avoid detection. The vast majority of sex offenders know that their behaviour is illegal and in order to offend have had to overcome their internal inhibitions. They may do this in a number of ways, such as developing cognitive distortions to justify and excuse their behaviour. They may also use alcohol or drugs as disinhibitors (as discussed in Factor 4) and then use cognitive distortions to blame the disinhibitors for the offending, rather than seeing it as a way of allowing themselves to behave in a way that they already wanted to. It is therefore important in treatment to focus on identifying and challenging distorted thinking, as discussed in Chapters 4, 5 and 6, to prevent them from progressing into a high-risk situation.

3 **Overcoming external inhibitions** Once the offender has overcome his internal inhibitions against carrying out the offence he must then set up a situation in which the offence can occur and overcome any external obstacles that may arise. This is akin to the planning and grooming phase of the assault cycle. Although it is possible that some offenders, especially young adolescents, may find themselves in a situation where they offend opportunistically, the vast majority of offenders create situations, such as offering to baby-sit or forming a relationship with a single parent in order to gain access to a child. The absence of the child's mother, which can be used as an excuse by the offender, may have been purposefully engineered in order to access the child. The focus for treatment is to develop a relapse prevention plan by helping the offender

to identify risk situations and appropriate methods of exiting safely from them. These issues are also relevant to work with the non-abusing parent, as described in Chapter 8.

4 **Overcoming the resistance of the child/victim**   The final precondition focuses on the methods the offender employs to overcome any resistance the victim may offer. As with the setting up of the situation in which abuse can occur, offenders can go to great lengths to ensure that they overcome the resistance of the victim. The grooming of the victim may involve developing a friendship with the child, using bribes of affection and gifts, threats or physical violence. Some offenders may target particular children who are perceived as being vulnerable in some way, possibly through poor parenting or previous sexual abuse. How an offender targets and grooms his victims provides vital information for child protection agencies and non-abusing parents to assist them in monitoring offenders in the longer term. The principal aims of treatment in this respect are to help the offender identify the ways in which he has abused his power and authority and to develop his empathy about the effects on his victims of his offending.

CONCLUSIONS

Whilst the multi-factorial models may be criticised on a number of issues, and do not provide a full explanation as to why all sex offenders offend, they are certainly more comprehensive and adequate than single-factor theories. It is likely that as more becomes known about sex offenders, it will be possible to develop more accurate models for different types of offenders. Although this review of the literature has been selective and each of the models outlined has limitations, collectively they provide a useful base from which to understand the behaviour of child sexual abusers and for planning assessment and treatment.

2 Context, constraints and considerations for practice

Tony Morrison

Understanding the context in which practice takes place is vital. It enables the practitioner to take proper account of the wide-ranging set of influences which bear upon their ability to be effective, including societal attitudes, legislation and organisational factors. Some, probably the majority, of these influences lie beyond the control of the practitioner, not least the acute resource shortages in health and welfare agencies. Nonetheless, if practitioners do not take such factors into account, intervention and treatment plans may be unrealistic and inappropriate, leading to failure and disillusionment. A particular danger in working with sex offenders is becoming overly responsible at a personal level for the success or failure of work with clients, because of the propensity of sex offenders to project onto others responsibility for their actions and feelings. Arguably the more significant influences in dealing with offenders' denial are not the individual skills of practitioners, but the impact on offenders of effective co-ordination between the child protection and criminal justice systems.

Whilst there are therefore factors which are beyond the control of the practitioner, there are many other factors to which practitioners working in this field can and should attend. These concern matters of philosophy, values, theoretical orientation, ethics, professional preparation and support. It is not sufficient to understand the research outlined in the previous chapter, or to seek to apply the practical models outlined in the following chapters, without first considering these issues. It is only by doing so that practitioners can properly equip themselves, and help to influence their agency to create conditions in which good practice in a turbulent world can flourish.

It is intended therefore that this chapter will be of use not only to practitioners working with adults or juveniles, but that it may also be a resource document or discussion paper at a managerial level. Many senior managers, whilst acknowledging in general terms the importance of this work, remain, through lack of practice experience, genuinely unclear about the philosophy and theoretical basis underpinning the management of sex offenders. This is even more pronounced where juvenile sex offenders are concerned.

If this work is to become properly integrated within the mainstream of agency philosophy and provision, managers and practitioners need to develop shared understandings about their rationale and approach, both within and between agencies. There are also implications that arise from working with sex offenders for work with other client groups involved in child protection and correctional work. Practitioners have a key role to play in making these links and developing organisational awareness and responsiveness to the management of sex offenders.

The chapter is divided into three sections. The first considers the organisational context of this work, looking at both intra- and interagency factors. The second section considers the impact of societal and legislative responses to sex offenders, with particular reference to the Children Act 1989, the Criminal Justice Act 1991, and the sentencing of offenders. The final section examines the philosophy of intervention, as well as theoretical and ethical factors.

ORGANISATIONAL CONTEXT

Development of sex offender treatment

Any discussion of context must begin with some reflection on the historical development of the field and its impact on the philosophy and approach to the task of managing sex offenders. Between 1983 and 1987, child protection registers showed an 800 per cent increase in the registration of children as a result of sexual abuse (Home Office, 1989). In the same period, prosecutions for sexual offences rose by only 17 per cent (Home Office, 1989). In other words, whilst the professional community was facing an explosion of demand to protect and care for the victims of sexual abuse, the criminal justice system appeared to be ineffective in identifying and controlling the offenders. Apart from a very limited amount of treatment being provided in NHS settings, services to sex offenders were almost non-existent until the later part of the 1980s.

It was thus not surprising, in the light of such figures, that a major impetus behind the rapid expansion of interest in services for sex offenders came from front-line professionals working in or alongside the child protection system. This was fuelled and informed by a succession of national conferences, the work of Ray Wyre and the Gracewell Clinic, and the establishment of NOTA, the National Association for the Development of Work with Sex Offenders. As a result, several key messages were disseminated into the professional system. Firstly research, particularly that of Abel *et al.* (1987), showed that the true extent of sexual offending is far greater and more complex than official figures reveal. Secondly, and more recently, adolescents have been found to account for up to a third of all sexual offending (Northern Ireland Research Team, 1991). Thirdly, sex offence specific programmes in North America appeared to show promising results to justify resourcing of intensive and long-term treatment (Marshall, Ward *et al.*, 1991).

The outcome was the rapid emergence in the late 1980s and early 1990s of mainly group work treatment programmes, predominantly aimed at male intra-familial sex offenders (Barker and Morgan, 1993). However, many of these programmes were run by practitioners outside normal working hours, in addition to their normal workload. Indeed, at the time of writing some still are. Such programmes were thus operating on the goodwill of motivated staff, without agency ownership, support, supervision, guidance or policy. The NCH report on children and young people who abuse other children summarised the position in 1992:

> Uncertainty about the legitimacy of the work and the complex consequences of denial combine to create great pressure on the member of staff. Management denial of the need to work with young abusers can leave staff isolated and unclear whether or not this is a legitimate area for them to be involved in.

One of the factors which has contributed to this lack of managerial ownership has been a tendency for work with sex offenders to be seen, unhelpfully, as being fundamentally distinct from work with other clients who, for example, have physically abused their children or who are involved in criminal activity.

This philosophical and theoretical abstraction reinforced the organisational isolation of this work within agencies. It also created difficulties, both for workers in being able to transfer skills and knowledge from previous practice to this field, and for managers feeling unable to offer proper supervision.

Agency and interagency context

In response to such concerns, there has been a growing recognition by government, and increasingly by agencies, of the need to create a proper organisational and interagency infrastructure for the work. In November 1990 the Home Secretary announced a major initiative for the treatment of sex offenders in prisons. There has also been an acceptance of the role which central government departments need to play in setting the context and framework for multi-agency work at a local level (Inspectorate of Probation, 1991). This was further reflected in the work of the Inter-Departmental Group on Child Abuse 'Strategic Statement on Working with Abusers' (1992), which set out the aims of government departments at a national level. These statements, taken with the Home Office paper, *Supervision of Sex Offenders* (1992), have provided a clear mandate and rationale for work with sexual offenders. They make clear that the overarching aim of work with offenders is the protection of victims.

Working Together under the Children Act 1989 (1991), also for the first time located the management of juvenile sex offenders within the child protection system:

> Work with adult abusers has shown that many of them begin committing their abusing acts during childhood or adolescence and that significant numbers have suffered from abusing acts themselves. It is therefore an important child protection function to ensure that such behaviour is treated seriously and is always subject to a referral to child protection agencies.

> (Para. 5.24)

Thus case conferences should be held not only on the victims of such offenders, but also on the young person.

Undoubtedly these are signs of progress, but practitioners will be only too aware of the constraints operating at ground level. Hallett and Birchall (1992) summarise these when they describe

> the atmosphere of chronic overstrain, unrealistic expectations of staff, desperately inadequate resources to cope with rapidly increasing reportage of cases and a limited fund of skills and knowledge confronting rising expectations that abuse should always be successfully managed.

Practitioners will be under no illusions, either, about the complexities and constraints to interagency collaboration. As Aiken (1975) comments, 'collaboration is a word which is overworked, underachieved and seldom defined.'

These difficulties are exacerbated by some of the feelings, dynamics and theoretical tensions involved in dealing with sexual abuse. The potential for the anger and distress felt by all involved to spill out in punitive responses, or to be suppressed via denial or collusion, is a real danger. When this happens, collaboration is threatened. Both agencies and individuals can unwittingly come to mirror or reflect in their dealings with each other, the dynamics of sexual abuse in which they are striving to intervene (Furniss, 1987). Secrecy, domination, denial, shame, victimisation and collusion within the professional network can all undermine colleague, supervisory and interagency relationships.

This, then, is part of the interagency context in which work with sex offenders is set. There are also a number of additional organisational factors which need to be addressed. They are included not because it is the responsibility of the practitioner to resolve them, but because the practitioner needs to understand and bring to the notice of managers organisational features that constrain practice. In mentioning these it is difficult to gauge the extent to which these are being addressed in different agencies and parts of the country. Certainly there has been considerable progress in some agencies and areas in providing managerial ownership and support. However, the overall picture remains very patchy. For some readers, therefore, what follows may describe a climate that no longer applies, whilst for others many of the problems may still be very real, especially for those working with juvenile offenders. (For a detailed description see NCH Report, 1992.) These are the principal factors:

1 **An absence of ownership at senior management level** This can be reflected in a lack of clear philosophy, policy and strategic planning for working with sex offenders. Under such conditions the work remains very largely the responsibility of interested practitioners and may be at odds with the agency's traditional value or policy base, for instance over matters such as confidentiality, or minimum intervention with juveniles.

2 **A lack of interagency arrangements** Area Child Protection Committees (ACPCs) in each local authority have responsibility for co-ordinating the response of agencies to child protection, and the management of sex offenders needs to be considered as part of this. Unfortunately current experience suggests that the degree to which ACPCs are attending to this area is very uneven. In the case of juvenile offenders there is no clear consensus across agencies as to the definition of what constitutes juvenile sexual offending, and there are tensions between police and social work agencies about the investigation of such referrals. Many areas are not holding conferences on juvenile offenders and in some cases they are being managed without any proper reference to child protection procedures (NCH, 1992). Whilst the guidance in *Working Together* is a start, it is plainly not sufficient, and overburdened agencies are unable to accommodate the resource-intensive demands of this emerging area of work.

3 **Absence of practice guidance** The sexually explicit and very intimate nature of work with sex offenders, and the strong feelings generated in those working with them, mean that the potential for defensive, voyeuristic or persecutory practice is high. The motivation for those working in this field may be variable and sometimes only partially acknowledged by the practitioner.

In such a practice environment, a lack of practice standards and ethical guidance is concerning. Managers are unable to exercise accountability, and clients, workers and agencies are vulnerable if, for example, complaints are made, or practice is thought to be unsatisfactory. It also hinders the development of the consistency and accountability in practice so necessary to gain judicial and public credibility.

4 **Inadequate supervisory arrangements** Few supervisors have experience of this work and many therefore feel understandably diffident about supervising their staff, especially in the absence of a policy framework. Supervisors themselves require support and training, as well as access to consultation over the management of cases. The Probation Inspectorate (1991) commented that 'some supervisors were not sufficiently aware that confronting sexual behaviour requires staff to examine their personal attitudes and behaviour, and indeed their relationships in a way that does not apply with other types of offender'. It is essential that supervisors understand and work with the gender issues which are provoked by this work, for both male and female staff. The dangers are that supervisors may either abandon staff when it comes to this area of work, or fail to understand its nature and the personal demands made on them.

5 **Shortage of facilities** Although there has been a rapid growth in the number of group treatment programmes for adult offenders, many practitioners still do not have access to a specific assessment or treatment facility at a local level. The majority of work is undertaken on an individual basis in the local office. Where juveniles in care are concerned, social services are faced with severe problems over placement in mixing victims and abusers in one setting. There is a need for a continuum of care, ranging from secure to community provision, which simply does not exist at present. A particular concern is the lack of knowledge, skills and resources in working with black offenders. This concern is amplified by the fact that black defendants in general experience discrimination within the criminal justice system. Grubin and Gunn (1990) found that black offenders were over-represented in their survey of rapists serving prison sentences. Practitioners thus find themselves in conflict. On the one hand it is essential to ensure that all offenders take appropriate responsibility for their offending behaviour, whilst on the other, it is important to protect clients from ethnic minority groups from unfair and discriminatory treatment by both criminal justice and child protection systems. However, as Gerrilyn Smith points out in Chapter 8, cross-cultural competence in the child protection field is very embryonic. White practitioners certainly report considerable difficulties in responding to black offenders, whilst the experience of

black practitioners over this issue has been barely discussed. As Cowburn and Wilson (1992) point out, such concerns have to be located within a more widespread concern about the overall negative experience of black staff and clients within welfare and judicial agencies. Whilst there is considerable cross-cultural consensus that sexual abuse is unacceptable and harmful (UN Convention on the Rights of the Child, 1989), we lack detailed knowledge, training and skills about cross-cultural meanings of sexuality, gender relationships and culturally sensitive ways of intervening.

All of these factors are further reflected and worsened when it comes to facilities for black offenders. Group treatment programmes are very largely staffed by white practitioners for offenders who are almost all white. Under such conditions it is not surprising that referrals to such programmes for black clients appear, anecdotally at least, to be so low. In addition there are problems where interpreting facilities are required. The demands on interpreters dealing with sexually explicit discussion, and trying to convey with precision processes such as cognitive distortions are extremely complex and emotionally fraught. Those who are asked to provide such a service require extensive support and training. Until more attention is paid to these issues, black offenders will be further disadvantaged by the lack of appropriate and accessible services.

It is vital that progress in tackling these organisational issues continues, for the potential consequences of not doing so are well known to practitioners:

It was the view of experienced and knowledgeable staff that those working with sex offenders are vulnerable because they have to make crucial judgements about risk . . . and confront denial after denial . . . The evidence from the inspection suggests that, if there is not sufficient training or support, some staff may well withdraw or collude with the offender's denial of responsibility.

(Probation Inspectorate, 1991)

These organisational factors have a direct bearing on practice. Whilst beyond his or her direct control, the practitioner may have varying degrees of influence in relation to them. Being aware of these factors is important in order to work with them in as effective a manner as possible, as well as to prevent practitioners feeling responsible for things that lie beyond their control.

Accepting that no setting is perfect, readers may find it valuable to consider the extent to which the framework presented below exists within their own setting. If there are deficits, how does this affect practice, staff development and morale? It is important to think about what alliances

Organisational building blocks

☐   evaluation of practice
☐   staff care policy and provision
☐   supervision and consultation
☐   resources and prioritisation of service delivery
☐   training for managers and practitioners
☐   policy and practice guidance
☐   philosophy of intervention
☐   structures for policy and practice development and leadership
☐   mandate and legitimisation for work with sex offenders
☐   recognition of the need to work with sex offenders

Figure 2.1 Organisational building blocks

within the agency or one's peer group could be mobilised to start addressing such areas.

Whatever influence practitioners may be able to exert, it is important to remember that it is the responsibility of managers to establish the organisational framework without which good practice cannot thrive. But as we turn our attention to the societal and legislative context in which agencies operate, it will become clear that there exist other factors which are themselves beyond the influence of even the most senior managers.

SOCIETAL AND LEGISLATIVE CONTEXT

Societal responses

Child abuse in general, and sexual abuse in particular, present a profound challenge to society. The 'discovery' and social response to child abuse over the past three decades have been accompanied by turbulent swings in public opinion, with professionals being accused, sometimes simultaneously, of either doing too little too late or too much too soon. Such societal ambivalence undermines professional confidence and hinders the emergence of a coherent response to child abuse.

In the case of sexual abuse, Olafson, Corwin and Summit (1993) have described societal responses in terms of 'cycles of discovery and suppression' in which

> the sexual abuse of children has repeatedly surfaced into public and professional awareness in the past century and a half, only to be re-suppressed by the negative reaction it elicits. The result has been a long history of cultural denial about sexual behaviour against children. As a society we behave somewhat like those victims who protect themselves

from their pain and terror by splitting off and sealing over all memory of childhood sexual traumas. There are some indications that this cultural dissociation is persisting in spite of substantial contemporaneous research on child sexual abuse.

The Cleveland affair represented a watershed in the UK's response to sexual abuse. However, the inquiry decided to seek no evidence about sex offenders, and that in one of the few references to the causes of sexual abuse, Professor Sir Martin Roth stated:

> In many cases, mothers play a role in the genesis of the sexual abuse of their daughters. From a normal daughter/father relationship in an isolated family, a bereaved husband may sometimes, not with any very great pathology in certain cases, slide, without any clearly formed intent, into a sexual relationship.

Such a statement, seeing the mother as blameworthy and the offender in the victim role, says much about the difficulty that professionals can have in confronting abusers with their responsibility.

Public responses to sex offenders have thus vacillated between over-tolerance and collusion on the one hand, and intolerance and repulsion on the other. The outcry about police and social work investigations into suspected cases in Cleveland in 1986, Rochdale in 1990 and Orkney in 1991, led to major inquiries. All these inquiries concluded that there had been major errors in the interviewing and management of children by both police and social workers. In some cases this was attributed to over-zealousness on the part of under-trained and poorly supervised interviewers. The late 1980s saw a formidable backlash from politicians, courts and the media. Critics, such as Wakefield and Underwager (1988), argued that sexual abuse was over-reported, especially in custody disputes, and that children make false allegations. The exposure of poor investigative practice together with the climate of backlash have resulted in an atmosphere of excessive caution on the part of child protection agencies about statutory intervention. Proving sexual abuse in the courts has become increasingly difficult.

In contrast, public reaction to cases such as that of Frank Beck, the residential social worker manager given a total of five life sentences for multiple sexual assaults on children in care, and more generally, to reports of sexual aggression outside the family, has been consistently punitive. The public are largely ignorant and at best ambivalent about the treatment of sex offenders. Whilst some believe that the only response should be punishment, others, whilst supportive of the idea of treatment, are not happy to have facilities within their own communities. The organised resistance, including the use of violence in the form of arson attacks, to attempts by the Gracewell Clinic to relocate their residential treatment facility have been a powerful testament to the public distaste for any constructive approach to the management of sex offenders. As one leading protester commented: 'We have been forced to think about issues we would rather not have faced. Our children are having their innocence taken away' (*Independent on Sunday*, 3 October, 1993).

In a climate that is increasingly hostile to offenders in general, there may be significant potential risks of a public backlash against all sex offender treatment, if there should be a serious and publicly exposed treatment failure. In Canada, following the assault and murder of a woman by an offender who was attending a residential treatment facility, a high-level inquiry about the future of all offender treatment was commissioned (Cormier, 1988). Olafson, Corwin and Summit (1993) conclude:

> It remains to be seen whether the current backlash will succeed in re-suppressing awareness [of sexual abuse] . . . If this occurs, it will not happen because child sexual abuse is peripheral to major social interests, but because it is so central, so that as a society we choose to reject our knowledge of it rather than make the changes in our thinking, our institutions and our daily lives that sustained awareness of child sexual victimisation demands.

As practitioners, we too need to consider the implications of working with sex offenders, in terms not only of our professional understanding of sexual abuse, but its implications both for the institutions in which we work and our own family and social relationships. Professional practice cannot be divorced from its wider implications in our daily lives.

Legislation

The Children Act 1989 and the Criminal Justice Act 1991 set the legislative framework for child protection and work with offenders in the 1990s. Both were reforming pieces of legislation intended to establish a new philosophy and approach to their respective areas of concern. The effects, both intended and unintended, of these Acts were still, in mid-1993, only beginning to become clear as the Appeal Court began to respond, particularly to the Children Act. It remains to be seen how far the Criminal Justice Act changes the response of the courts to sex offenders. Serious problems remain in the management of sexual offence cases by the criminal courts, due to the Appeal Court Guidelines on sentencing (which are discussed below), judicial attitudes to sexual offences, delays in processing such cases and the constraints operating on prosecuting authorities.[1]

The Children Act 1989

This Act's central emphasis on partnership with families – working wherever possible without recourse to statutory intervention – and its preventative rationale do not fit easily with the management of child sexual abuse. Establishing viable partnerships on a voluntary basis with sex offenders is highly problematic, given their propensity to deny and minimise the true nature of their offending behaviour, their distorted thinking, and the compulsive and damaging nature of their actions. Additionally their manipulative behaviour within families gives rise to concern about the freedom of all other family members to work openly and freely with child protection agencies when sexual abuse has been disclosed. As Sgroi (1982) has argued:

> The track record of persuading perpetrators of sexual abuse to undergo voluntary therapy is abysmal. Perpetrators rarely remain in an effective treatment programme when the pressure to participate slackens. Why do we ignore the compelling evidence that an authoritative incentive to change his or her behaviour is absolutely essential for the adult perpetrator of sexual abuse?

There are particular difficulties in decisions about contact between offenders and victims. The Act makes the presumption (s. 44) that when children are removed from home, there should be contact with parents. However, as Salter (1992) puts it, 'when the touching stops, the [psychological] abuse may not.' Summit's *Accommodation Syndrome* (1983) has described how victims internalise the abuser's distorted messages, believe that they are to blame for being abused and then become psychologically entrapped and accommodated to the abuser. Such 'groomed' children, without treatment and the full support of a non-abusing parent, are highly vulnerable to continuing psychological abuse, resulting in retraction if contact is prematurely re-established.

Children want the abuse to stop, but at the same time often do not want to lose their father-figure. The Act's emphasis on the rights of children and the importance of involving them in decision-making processes cannot be ignored in matters of sexual abuse. There are many unresolved questions as to what in practice it means to take the wishes and feelings of children into account. We are as yet unclear as to the degree of prominence a child's wishes should play in deciding questions of contact or rehabilitation. The question remains, however, as to how impaired the views and wishes of sexually abused children may be. As Eldridge observes (1991), 'We do not make things better by colluding with the voice of the offender when it is coming from the victim's mouth, rather than the offender's.' There is a critical need for assessment, not just of the offender, but for comprehensive family assessment, if the best decisions are to be made. Such an assessment will need to consider not only the strength of a child's attachment to their abuser, but equally the nature of it. A child may be strongly but negatively attached. Salter (1992) describes 'abuse-distorted attachments' as normal affectionate attachment bonds which have been distorted by the dynamics of abuse, and where the child seeks proximity with the offender at any cost. She lists the following preconditions in terms of the progress made by the child, aside from the offender's work, for contact to take place:

1 a reduction in the victim's thinking errors so that he or she does not minimise, encapsulate or rationalise the abuse;
2 he or she is sufficiently assertive to say 'no';
3 he or she is willing to say no;
4 he or she has a bond with the mother which is sufficient to disclose;
5 traumatic flashbacks have disappeared or markedly decreased;
6 he or she has a victim alert list based on some understanding of the offender's cycle.

(Clearly the above assumes that the child is of sufficient age to participate in such work. Where a younger/pre-verbal child is involved, much more will depend on the progress of the non-abusing parent. This is discussed in Chapter 8.)

Salter concludes by stating that too often all that is required for abused children to be returned home, is that someone believes that the mother will protect the child from being physically assaulted again. As a result, Salter concludes, many victims are living in households where they are constantly affected with traumatic flashbacks.

Unfortunately one of the unintended consequences of the recent increase in treatment programmes for offenders, is that this may result in situations where this is the only treatment work being undertaken, with no treatment service being available for children or the non-abusing parent. Anecdotal evidence at least suggests that treatment provision for abused children is woefully inadequate, perhaps covering less than 10 per cent of sexually abused children placed on child protection registers. Treatment services for non-abusing parents are probably even scarcer. Children cannot be protected by working only with the offender. If victims are to become survivors, both they and their non-abusing parent will need as much help and effort to recover, as the offender will do to change his behaviour.

With the majority of offenders, who are not prosecuted, an immediate problem following disclosure is how to secure the offender's, rather than the victim's, removal, from the home. If this is not done, both the children and the non-abusing parent may continue to be psychologically dominated by the offender, limiting the prospects for any effective treatment or preventative work. Removal of the victim from the home does not control the offender. Unfortunately the Children Act confers very little power on the local authority in this respect. Whilst social services may assist (s. 17) materially with an offender moving out of the home, they cannot compel him to do so. The Orkney report (Clyde,1992) recommended that consideration be given in child care legislation to provision for removing the offender. One of the main benefits of prosecution is that a conviction, followed by a probation order, with added conditions, can enable the supervising officer to compel the offender to leave the home.

Overall, then, the Children Act conveys relatively limited powers to control the offender who is not convicted, without removing the victim from home. This position was reinforced by an Appeal Court judgment in *Re P (Minors) Nottingham C.C.* (1993), in which the Appeal Court quashed a prohibited steps order made by a lower court designed to prevent a father, who had sexually abused one daughter over a lengthy period, having contact with the other children in the family. The judges criticised social services for failing to pursue care proceedings as a method of protecting the children, and instead pursuing an application for a section 8 order to control his contact with the family.

The problems faced by social services in having responsibility, without having either the powers or resources to manage sex offenders, were also highlighted during this case. They were unable to fund a place for the father to receive treatment on a residential basis at the Gracewell Clinic, stating in evidence that

> In this department we are very much aware of the great need for therapeutic intervention and counselling with men such as this. We experience on a daily basis the risks posed to young people by such men, and keenly feel the dearth of resources to deal with Schedule 1 offenders.

It is also doubtful how far the Children Act allows courts to order parents to participate in treatment, except where children are subject to care orders, and treatment for the parents is made a condition of rehabilitation being considered. The other means might be through a condition which can be attached to a supervision order, directing the parents to cooperate with the child's supervising officer.

With regard to juvenile sex offenders, the main effect of the Act has been to end criminal care orders at a point where, some would argue, a real purpose had been found for them. This means that a juvenile offender can now only be made subject of a care order if it can be shown that he or she is suffering 'significant harm', as shown by their offending behaviour, rather than because of the harm they cause others. Although juvenile offenders have by definition of their behaviour shown evidence of impaired development, this measure may undermine the young person's sense of responsibility for his or her own behaviour. The alternative, a supervision order, suffers from the absence of meaningful sanctions in the event of token or non-compliance. The only real sanction, that of substituting a care order, thus almost certainly depends on reoffending. Finally it remains to be seen whether Schedule 3 of the Act will enable the parents of juvenile offenders, so crucial to treatment work but often very reluctant to participate, to be directed to cooperate with supervisors in treatment work.

The Criminal Justice Act 1991

This Act has produced major changes for practice both in the courts and the probation service, much of which are centred on the concepts of seriousness and restriction of liberty. It lays down one primary purpose of sentencing which is punishment, and restriction of liberty as the single measure of punishment to be applied across the whole range of community and custodial sentences.

There are, however, special provisions in the case of violent or sexual offences where the court can pass longer sentences where this is considered necessary for the protection of the public. The Act also gives the court power to require that sex offenders receive longer post-release supervision. Balanced against this, probation orders are now a sentence under the Act, with additional conditions available, giving the possibility of more non-custodial sentences for sex offenders, where custody is not seen as necessary.

As far as young offenders are concerned, the Act introduces Youth Courts to deal with offenders aged ten to 17 years. Probation orders can be made from 16 years and may be combined with community service orders, attendance centre orders, or curfew orders. For offenders under 16 years the Act seeks to emphasise parental responsibility for the behaviour of the offender. This may have unpredictable consequences. The juvenile may be able to offset his responsibility, and parents may understandably reject the idea that they are to blame for their adolescent's sexual behaviour.

The Act also introduced Pre-Sentence Reports (PSRs) which are to assist the court in deciding between custodial and community sentences. In the case of sex offenders this will include an assessment of the risk of serious harm that the offender might pose, together with a clear presentation about the aims, range and likely effectiveness of treatment options. The fact that the Act allows reference to prior convictions and evidence of previous similar patterns of behaviour (s.29 (2)) gives those writing reports on sex offenders particular scope to identify and comment on offenders' distorted thinking and manipulative behaviours. This should ensure that the court has a clear picture about the offender's responsibility and the ways in which he gained access and coerced the victim into the abusive situation or relationship.

In the light of the Appeal Court guidelines for sentencing, discussed below, practitioners will also need to be clear as to what aggravating and mitigating factors there may be, which should be discussed in the PSR. Interestingly research by McColl and Hargreaves (1992) on a sample of social enquiry reports on adult male sex offenders found that a significant proportion of probation officers found difficulty in attributing culpability. 'Those who appeared to accept offender explanations or were persuaded that other factors in the offender's circumstances made his actions more comprehensible, suggested lower culpability.' Cowburn and Wilson (1992) comment:

> It would appear to be particularly important that Probation Services make decisions on what these aggravating or mitigating factors may be. Any policy or professional decision will originate from a value base concerned with sexual violence. Services and professional bodies need to consider whether they will endorse or collude with the values of male domination and thus minimise and dismiss sexual violence. To adopt the latter will mean that there can be few mitigating factors where sex offences are concerned. This may prove a difficult position for many probation officers to take, when, traditionally the probation service has sought to ameliorate the harshness of the criminal justice process.

We therefore turn now to look in more detail at the response of the criminal justice system to sexual offenders.

Reporting and sentencing trends

Home Office statistics show that between 1980 and 1990, reports of sexual offences increased from 21,107 to 29,044 per year, the greatest increase being for rapes. Approximately 16 per cent of all reported sexual offences concerned alleged offences against children. However, what has remained fairly even throughout this period has been the consistently high proportion of these reported crimes which have been 'cleared up'. In other words, in the vast majority of these cases the police have been able to identify the person responsible.

Despite the high 'clear-up' rates, the proportion of offenders either cautioned or prosecuted has been much lower. In 1990 3,300 offenders were cautioned, of whom 800 were between 17 and 20 years and 1,000 between 14 and 16 years. Whilst a small proportion may have been cautioned for technical offences in the context of a consenting relationship, the majority were for abusive acts. Indeed more young males in the 17 to 20 years group were cautioned (800) than found guilty (700) for sexual offences.

The Home Office (1990a) Circular on Cautioning (59/90) states:

> Cautioning is an efficient effective and economic response to offending behaviour which is relatively minor, opportunistic and transient . . . . As far as the offence is concerned the most serious offences are not seen as suitable for caution nor those where the victim has suffered significant harm or loss.

Clearly sexual offending does cause significant harm, and is one of several reasons why cautioning has limitations for sex offences. As cautioning must be unconditional, it cannot be used as a mandate to engage the offender in treatment, nor as a sanction if he should drop out of treatment undertaken on a voluntary basis. Nevertheless, in view of the problems involved in prosecution described below, it would be unreasonable to conclude that there is no place for cautioning. One of the key factors, however, is to ensure that juvenile offenders receive both proper assessment and treatment. The NCH (1992) report on young offenders concluded that programmes must be available on both a legally mandated and a voluntary basis. Given some of the problems with prosecution, and the limits of the current arrangements for cautioning, there is a strong argument for the development of diversion policies based on a plea of guilt, and a much strengthened conditional cautioning system, with the sanction to prosecute the offender in the event of non-compliance with treatment.

In 1990, 6,500 offenders were found guilty. Put another way, this meant that in that year there was a less than one in four chance that a reported sex offence would result in a conviction. The principal sentences were as follows:

Immediate custody	2,200
Fine	1,900
Probation order	900
Absolute or conditional discharge	700
Supervision order	100
Community service	100

(Home Office, 1991)

Despite the gradual decrease in the use of fines, it is still of considerable concern that an offender is twice as likely to be fined as to be put on probation or supervision. The largest group are those given an immediate custodial sentence. However, whilst a proportion of these are offenders too dangerous to be managed in the community, the anti-therapeutic effects of incarceration on the majority of sex offenders cannot be ignored if the goal is the prevention of further abuse. As the Woolfe Inquiry commented:

> When Rule 43 prisoners are subject to assaults or worse this makes them feel, with justification, that they are the victims. This focuses their attention on their own condition and away from what they have done to their victims. These offenders must be required to confront their criminal conduct.
>
> (Woolfe Report, 1991)

In response to this and other reports, the Government announced a major prison service treatment programme for sex offenders, initially targeting all inmates serving four years or more. However, implementation of this programme has varied widely. There are also questions about the management of at least half the sex offender population who serve sentences of less than four years. Many of these will return to their local communities or families, having had no treatment. They will be subject to a period of supervision, but many having served their time inside are very resistant to undertaking treatment on release. In relation to this group, many would argue that a probation order with an intense period of community-based treatment is likely to be more effective in reducing further offending, than a short prison sentence without treatment.

Prosecution: benefits and limitations

In the light of these trends in reporting and sentencing it is not surprising that there has been considerable debate as to the benefits or otherwise of prosecution. Different issues have been raised in respect of adult and juvenile offenders. Broadly speaking, advocates of a prosecution-oriented approach have argued on both moral and therapeutic grounds that appropriate court-ordered disposals offer the following potential benefits:

1 protection of the victim;
2 protection of the community;
3 ensuring complete investigation of the complaint;
4 demonstration in public that sexual abuse is a criminal act and is serious;
5 holding the offender publicly accountable for his actions;
6 determining consequences for the offender's actions;
7 supportimg victim's rights and reducing minimisation and denial by offender;
8 evaluating the need and potential for treatment;
9 enhancing the offender's motivation to change;

10   assuring continued treatment;
11   providing for follow-up and relapse prevention work;
12   documenting a record of offending.

(US National Task Force Report, 1988)

Those supporting these arguments see sexual abuse as a serious crime and believe that offenders require external pressure to face up to the extent of their behaviour and to enter and sustain treatment. They also see prosecution as an important way of validating the victim's experience. However, whilst dissenters from this position would not, in the main, wish to see sexual abuse decriminalised, they argue that the experience of the criminal justice system in reality delivers few of the benefits and several serious disadvantages. Their principal concerns are that:

1   the trauma for many child witnesses associated with giving evidence is abusive and outweighs the advantages of even a successful prosecution;
2   the distress or 'failure' of the child in the witness box can result in the collapse of the prosecution case, leaving the victim even more powerless in relation to the abuser;
3   prosecution cannot guarantee protection of the community unless the offender is contained in security for life;
4   sentencing does not necessarily reinforce the offender's responsibility if, for instance, he is fined, or worse, discharged after being found guilty;
5   the court process and judges' comments can minimise the victim's experience or even convey the message that the victim was to blame;
6   the lack of suitable assessment and treatment facilities means that prosecution does not guarantee there is a complete investigation of the complaint or that prosecution will lead to treatment;
7   in the case of juvenile offenders there is concern about the potentially damaging effects of being drawn into the criminal justice system, especially if this results in a period in custody where mixing with other criminals may deepen the young offender's criminality;
8   concern about the labelling of juvenile offenders with Schedule 1 status whilst still in a formative stage of development;
9   the family of the offender may not want prosecution and may therefore align with the offender against the professionals, and become resistant to engaging in treatment;
10   the threat of prosecution may decrease the willingness of the offender to be open with assessors, fearing increased penalties in court if he admits the full extent of his offending behaviour.

Whether or not prosecution is effective either in protecting victims or ensuring an offender's compliance with treatment, depends on the degree of mutual understanding and collaboration between child protection and criminal justice systems. However, as Wattam (1993) has noted, the driving force behind amendments in the Criminal Justice Act for vulnerable witnesses has been the needs of the criminal justice system, rather than those of the child protection system or children. There remains therefore serious concern about the experience of abused children in the criminal courts. Without further reforms, including the full implementation of the Pigot Report, the value of prosecution, whilst in theory beneficial, will in practice remain very mixed. As David Jones (1993) has commented:

> Any perceived primacy of the prosecution process over the welfare of the child needs to be countered, but there will always be tension between the two. If the Criminal Justice Act means that more children give evidence, it should not mean that more children are harmed by our intervention process. If the tension becomes unbearable, it is the system that will have to change not the children.

In the mean time, whatever the individual views of the practitioner, professionals encountering suspected cases of child sexual abuse have to report such cases to the statutory authorities. It is then up to the Crown Prosecution Service to decide whether or not to prosecute. In the case of juveniles, Juvenile Liaison Panels will determine whether to recommend cautioning or prosecution. Practitioners may be relieved that they do not have to take such decisions. Indeed it is very important that practitioners who assess or treat sex offenders have no role in determining their guilt or otherwise; it is the courts who do this. Nevertheless, the provision of a risk assessment report, particularly in assisting Juvenile Panels, is very important, as the criminal charge on its own is a poor indicator of risk, and thus of whether prosecution is indicated.

However, the practitioner is left with many questions about how the criminal justice system works to protect children from sexual abuse, and how to best influence it as a report writer, witness or treatment provider. Some understanding therefore of both how and why the courts deal with sex offenders is thus of great importance. To gain some insight into this, we can examine the Court of Appeal guidelines on the sentencing of sex offenders.

Appeal Court guidelines for sentencing sex offenders

These were laid down in the Appeal Court by Lord Chief Justice Lane in 1988 (see the Appendix to this book). They remain in force regardless of the Criminal Justice Act until further Appeal Court rulings are made. In a critique of these guidelines Yates (1990) argues they are based on a number of erroneous assumptions about the experience of victims and the dynamics of offending. To summarise, her main criticisms are:

1 there is an assumption in them that sexual abuse is not necessarily harmful, arising from the fact that far too little evidence is sought by the court as to the harm suffered by the victim and that longer-term effects may not be apparent at the point of sentence;
2 there is an assumption that older girls may consent or even enjoy the abuse, unless they show evidence of being subject to overt forms of threat and coercion;
3 the offender's power, through a position of trust and authority, to coerce children very subtly, and without overt threats, into abusive situations is not acknowledged;
4 the guidelines attribute partial blame to the victim by failing to distinguish between the child's behaviour, which may have become sexualised, as for instance in the case of children previously abused, and responsibility for the offence. They imply that blame can be laid with the victim, because he or she is sexualised, for the offender's inability to control his sexual urges. Male sexual urges are thus by implication seen as uncontrollable;
5 the model of sexual abuse underlying these guidelines is a family dysfunction one. In support of this, Yates quotes the following from Lord Lane:

> If one can properly decide any kind of 'incest' as the 'ordinary' type of case it will be one where the sexual relationship between husband and wife has broken down; the father has probably resorted to excessive drinking and the eldest daughter is gradually, by way of familiarities, indecent acts and suggestions made the object of the father's frustrated sexual inclinations.

The responsibility for the offending is thus laid at the door of a broken marriage, alcohol, sexual frustration and the child's promiscuous presentation. Such a model not only fails to address the full weight of the offender's responsibility for his actions, but also fails to explain the position of male victims.

The experience to date, therefore, of the criminal justice process in responding to sexual offending has been equivocal, to say the least. It is not surprising in the light of the above that practitioners continue to find examples of sentences and judges' comments which collude with the offenders' minimisations and distortions. However, it is important that practitioners are aware of these guidelines if they are to work effectively and knowledgeably with courts, both in protecting children and in managing offenders. Too often, child protection agencies and sentencers are unable to communicate properly because each perceives the other as not understanding their own roles, value systems, constraints and powers.

If the criminal courts in particular are to play a more constructive role in the management of sex offenders, then there will need to be a far greater effort to bridge this gap. Despite the improvements brought about by the Criminal Justice Act in protecting child witnesses, there is still a long way to go whilst the levels of understanding by many sentencers about sexual abuse remain uninformed, and in some cases, untouched by the accounts of victims as to the reality of sexual aggression.

In this organisational and legislative environment practitioners managing such cases may be helped by keeping the following in mind: first, it is the offender, not the worker, who was responsible for the abuse; second it is the offender, not the worker, who is responsible for not reoffending; third, managers are responsible for allocating or not allocating resources to do the job and recognising that a single worker cannot manage both victim and abuser; finally effective work with offenders can be undertaken on an individual basis in a local office by local practitioners given reasonable training, access to consult- ancy and managerial support for co-working.

THE CONTEXT FOR PRACTICE

Having explored factors which lie for the most part beyond the immediate control of the practitioner, this section focuses on those aspects to which the practitioner should attend if s/he is to prepare properly for work with sex offenders and to be effective. Practitioners who are equipped solely with research about the extent of sexual offending, commitment and enthusiasm, are ultimately unlikely to be effective in their practice. Matters of philosophy, values, theoretical orientation and ethics all require consideration. Whilst these are of importance to all areas of work, there are a number of particular consequences in this field if they are not thought through. Personal attitudes and attributes are also very relevant, and these are discussed in Chapter 9.

Common practitioner concerns

At the start of this chapter the tendency for this work to be perceived as fundamentally distinct from other related areas of work was mentioned. This has perhaps been fuelled by the language used by those working with sex offenders. Terms such as 'grooming', and 'sexual assault cycle', together with a focus on cognitive and behavioural approaches can be perceived as being elitist, jargonised and North American. Whilst some of these dangers are common to all new fields of work, the mystique and abstraction attached to this work has had a particularly unfortunate effect in a field concerned with a taboo area such as sexual deviancy. At its worst, those working with sex offenders have reported their peers or managers speculating suspiciously as to their motivation for this field, and feeling alienated from them. As one brave colleague declared, 'The myth I want to explode is that there is something wrong with my sex life that makes me want to do this work.'

It is the fact that we are dealing explicitly with deviant sexuality that gives this work a particular and deeply personal salience for practitioners. Looked at in this way, the difference between working with sex offenders and other offenders lies much less in the distinctiveness of sex offenders as a group of clients, than in what practitioners and managers bring on a personal level to this work. It is, in other words, much more to do with 'us' than 'them'. Perhaps there has been a need to project onto these clients aspects of sexuality that all of us find difficult to acknowledge?

Practitioners new to this field have reported a variety of concerns, including: being 'contaminated' by their clients; failing to prevent re-offending; being unable to separate the abusive behaviour from the person; not having the skills to work with these clients; colluding; losing control of therapeutic sessions; and personal sexual and psychological vulnerability. The consequences can be practice which is defensive, over-controlling, unempathic, and inconsistent, with practitioners unable to use or adapt existing knowledge and skills. The image is of a 'cordon sanitaire' operating between the practitioner and the client. Although understandable, many of these problems stem from a failure to integrate this work with other practice experience, insufficient training and inadequate philosophical and theoretical preparation. It is to these aspects that we now turn.

Preparing for practice

Philosophy of intervention

To work with sexual abuse and sexual offenders, practitioners need to consider their value base. How do they understand sexual abuse? How are its causes construed? Is offending a matter of individual pathology, or a manifestation of behaviour along the continuum of 'normal' male sexuality? What are the societal roots of sexual violence and the conditions which encourage and sanction possessive and objectifying male attitudes and behaviour towards women and children? As Juliet Darke (1990) observes:

> Although the existence of gender inequities is no longer disputed, the cultural insistence on perpetuating these disparities and, therefore, male

dominance, is rarely acknowledged. To this end we socialise males to be aggressive, to devalue women, and to relate to others in minimally empathic ways. Either way, sexual violence will end when men no longer have the power to define what and who the problem is.

Practitioners cannot be value-free in this field. They need to develop, both individually and corporately, a value base to their work. The following is based on work by Anna Salter (1988).

1 Sexual assault is always unacceptable and should be investigated as a crime.
2 Sexual assault is damaging to the victim.
3 Sexual assault results from an intention on the part of the offender to seek both sexual and emotional gratification from the victim.
4 Sexual assault represents an abuse of power.
5 The overarching aim of intervention is to protect victims and potential victims.
6 Intervention must be based on the offender taking full responsibility for the feelings, thoughts and behaviour which support his offending. Male sexual arousal is controllable.
7 Where it is in the victim's interests, sex offenders should be prosecuted.
8 The goal of intervention is to ensure that sex offenders can control their behaviour so that they do not reoffend or sexually abuse others.
9 The management of offenders requires a co-ordinated response involving criminal justice and child protection agencies.
10 In the longer term the prevention of sexual offences needs to address the sex role expectations of males in our society.

Theoretical orientation: change and treatment effectiveness

The history of work with sex offenders has included a range of approaches, from individual psychotherapy, family therapy and chemical therapy through to, more recently, cognitive and behavioural therapies with an emphasis on group treatment. As Barker and Morgan (1993) found in the UK, the main elements of adult offender treatment are fairly consistent; these are described in Chapters 3, 4, 5 and 6. With juveniles, though, there is less consensus (NCH, 1992). However, agreement about treatment components may not signify an underlying clarity of thinking as to what individual practitioners actually believe or understand about the processes of change in human behaviour. It is very revealing when practitioners are invited to explain their own beliefs about the process of change and to identify what they specifically do in working with their clients to promote change. Practitioners need to think this through before establishing treatment programmes.

There can also be disastrous effects on co-work when conflicting beliefs about change collide in the middle of a therapeutic session, as when one person's 'confrontation' is perceived by their colleague as persecution.

Some practitioners, such as psychologists, will have received specific therapeutic training as part of their professional training. For others, not-ably social work trained staff, this cannot be assumed. Indeed the use of the term 'therapist' would on the whole be alien. Moreover staff such as those working in residential establishments may not be qualified and may have had almost no training in treatment methods. It is a point of heated debate as to whether staff should be accredited as service providers in this, or indeed other, forms of child protection work, and at present this does not appear to be likely. Nevertheless, all staff offering intervention programmes need a variety of knowledge and skills, not only about sex offenders but also in general coun-selling and treatment work, as well as in legal and organisational considerations.

In many cases it is this very emphasis on changing behaviour and on clear outcomes that attracts practitioners to this field, in contrast to what they perceive to be the organisational emphasis on the less precise and less rewarding areas of service delivery with their emphasis on packages and throughput. Work with sex offenders can offer an exciting developmental opportunity in a difficult area of work. However, if practitioners are to practice effectively, they will need to be able to relate prior knowledge, research, skills and confidence to their new work. This will be greatly assisted if the close links between sexual offending and other forms of persistent and serious offending, and the link with addictive behaviours can be seen. Research from these areas can inform our work with sex offenders.

In recent years the correctional field has seen a resurgence of faith in correctional treatment. This renewed optimism has arisen from a number of very large-scale studies of treatment programmes which have been able to identify a number of effective intervention techniques (Andrews *et al.*, 1990). McIvor (1990) summarises these as being programmes that:

1 are likely to target high-risk offenders;
2 target offence behaviours or behaviours closely associated with it;
3 are likely to be community based;
4 have a cognitive and behavioural focus;
5 are clearly structured, based on proven theoretical methods and use clear, more directive approaches;
6 show clear planning and deliver as planned – have high 'treatment integrity';
7 are delivered by staff who are trained and committed to the models being used.

(McIvor, 1990)

The overall message from these studies is that some things work with some offenders. Roberts (1991), reviewing work on serious and persistent offenders, proposes four levels of intervention which need to be provided in community-based programmes:

1 **Specific offending behaviour components** This would include the work described in detail in Chapters 3 and 4 on the sexual assault cycle, looking at the sequence of events, thoughts, feelings and actions surrounding the assault, an analysis of patterns of offending over time, and ways of changing these behaviours. This addresses individual responsibility and the gratification obtained through offending.

2 **Offending associated behaviour components** These include anger control and alcohol abuse and other addictive problems. These contribute to the offender's poor coping style and increase the risks of offending. Again, analysis of their role in offending is required, together with the teaching of alternative coping strategies.

3 **Presenting problems brought by the client**, and work on resolving/moderating these. This will involve tackling interrelated factors of environmental stress and disadvantage such as unemployment, problems with housing, poverty and breakdowns in family relationships leading to isolation and the loss of positive social influences.

4 **Community reintegration components** These are designed to strengthen a non-criminal lifestyle, and to provide reintegration opportunities within the community. Examples include work on adult education, leisure, housing, and employment needs.

The strength of Robert's model is in its recognition of the multi-causal nature of offending, including sexual offending, and its recognition therefore of the need for multifaceted intervention programmes. Obviously each offender needs assessment as to the particular programme he requires, as sex offenders, no less than other offenders, are not a homogeneous group. In the past, work with sexual offenders has been criticised for failing to deal with the offence-specific components. It is important, however, that the corrective does not now lead to practice which ignores the other levels, even though they will not all be needed in every case, nor be delivered within one programme.

Finally, from the addiction field, Prochaska and Di Clemente (1982) have devised a comprehensive model of change, shown in Figure 2.2, based on work with smokers. Change can only start once the individual is in contemplation, accepting that they are part of both the origin and the solution to their problems. The four phases of change (contemplation, action, maintenance and lapse) are preceded by the pre-contemplation stage. It is at this latter point particularly that the skills of motivational interviewing (Miller, 1983) are most needed in moving the offender on to the first stage of change, contemplation. Whilst offenders are in the pre-contemplation phase, blaming others, denying their own responsibility, or simply unaware of the need to change, no change is possible. Pre-contemplation is thus the point at which initial assessment takes place in order to ascertain the individual's willingness to accept responsibility and the prognosis for change. During the contemplation phase the goal is to help the individual face the consequences of their actions, understand options for the future and come to believe in the possibility that they can change. Only at this point can a valid therapeutic contract for change be made. It may well take a considerable amount of work to get to this point, whatever the strength of any external mandate on the offender.

In the action stage the focus is on rehearsing new ways of thinking, behaving and feeling. Indeed all personal change is essentially a combination of these three basic processes. However, the accent is on trying things out in safe settings based on modelling, instruction or problem-solving techniques. Assuming progress, the next stage, maintenance, occurs when the new behaviours become internalised and generalised across different situations. They do not now depend on the presence of the therapist, and become consolidated and owned by the individual as part of themselves.

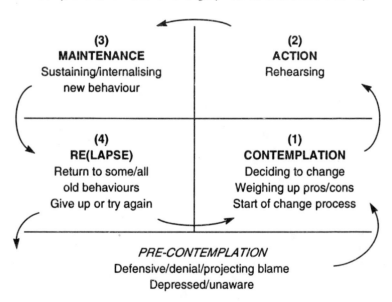

Comprehensive Model of Change (Prochaska and Di Clemente)

(3)
MAINTENANCE
Sustaining/internalising
new behaviour

(2)
ACTION
Rehearsing

(4)
RE(LAPSE)
Return to some/all
old behaviours
Give up or try again

(1)
CONTEMPLATION
Deciding to change
Weighing up pros/cons
Start of change process

PRE-CONTEMPLATION
Defensive/denial/projecting blame
Depressed/unaware

Figure 2.2 Prochaska and Di Clemente's comprehensive model of change

It is through this process that the client's sense of self-efficacy is increased.

The model proposes, however, that under stress, especially unpredictable stress, there may be the temptation to 'lapse', or there can be 'relapse', when the old behaviour pattern reappears. The relapse may lead to a loss of all or most of the treatment gains, resulting in a 'giving up', and a return to pre-contemplation. Alternatively in the case of a 'lapse', the client realises the dangers of sliding further back, tells himself that all is not lost, and seeks help urgently from friends, family or professionals. He thereby returns to the contemplation stage, which may lead to further treatment work. Because the possibility of relapse is anticipated in this model, relapse prevention forms an important part of the treatment as a way of forestalling such dangers. This is very important in the case of sex offenders.

One of the benefits of this model is that it integrates verbal and behavioural processes of change, such as consciousness raising, catharsis and insight at the contemplation stage, with action and contingency management techniques in the latter stages. It also suggests that successful change requires not just behavioural change but a restructuring of a person's thinking about themselves.

Ethical basis to practice

Because of the potential dangers inherent in all interventions, all forms of treatment should be underpinned by ethical principles. In this field, the strong feelings and personal issues generated make this all the more necessary, as Michael Sheath (1990) astutely observes:

> The attraction of overtly confrontational interviews, especially for male workers are manifold, and probably explain why the approach has gained popularity so quickly ... and I have to admit that my initial work with sex offenders was designed to give them as hard a time as possible. Since nonce-bashing was denied to me, I learnt the technique of the confrontational interview.

Unfortunately at present ethical guidance is not generally available. However, with the growth of programmes, the need for such guidance is pressing. Whatever an offender has done, this does not permit systems or individual practitioners to treat him as if he had forfeited his basic civil liberties.

Those wishing to undertake therapeutic work with offenders need to ask themselves whether they have compassion for their clients. They may at times also feel anger, distress and revulsion over the behaviour of offenders, or on behalf of the victim. But compassion, which is entirely different to collusion, is essential in forming effective therapeutic relationships. There has to be a fundamental respect for the dignity of the client as a human being, notwithstanding the fact that workers may be clear about and confrontative towards the offender's unacceptable behaviour. In recent times it has become fashionable to contrast traditional counselling ethics and the approach taken in working with sex offenders. Ross (1990) says: 'A new discipline of sexual aggression intervention has developed over the last decade utilising a very interventionist philosophy.' He describes the major differences with traditional mental health approaches as being:

1 a view that coerced participation in treatment can be effective if, over time, the offender becomes internally motivated to stop offending;
2 a view that insight has a less significant role in the change process than educational and cognitive and behavioural interventions;
3 that sex offenders should not be offered the same degree of confidentiality as other clients, as their behaviour needs to be monitored on an informed basis in many different settings outside the office;
4 that the helper role should not be seen as being in conflict with the social control role;
5 that the worker should accept the need to become involved in the criminal justice system because they are dealing with offenders who ignore the rights of others;
6 the need to recognise and utilise the offender's anxieties in order to facilitate disclosure, rather than seeking to put their client at ease in the interviewing situation;
7 that the roles of adversary and ally are always balanced in this non-traditional interviewing approach.

Ross also stresses the need to use the least restrictive option commensurate with the need to protect victims, in providing treatment for the offender. Finally he states that the offender should be given every possible opportunity to engage in treatment, before they are labelled as completely uncooperative.

Three core concepts in ethical intervention are informed consent, the nature of voluntariness, and confidentiality. Manning *et al.* (1992), as part of their preparations for an adolescent offenders' programme in Melbourne, considered these issues in some detail and concluded that clients have rights to:

1 the best possible treatment;
2 a second opinion;
3 information about the nature and length of the programme, both verbally and in writing;

4 complain about and/or to withdraw from treatment (assuming that the consequences of doing so are clear);
5 have their religious, cultural and language needs respected.

Following from the above, they argue that practitioners have the following obligations:

1 to brief referrers that professional ethics do not permit compulsory treatment for sex offenders (i.e. treatment against their will);
2 to carefully examine the identifiable sources of influence on clients as to their decisions to undergo or refuse treatment;
3 to ensure that the offender gives informed consent in writing to treatment after the risks and benefits have been explained, the alternatives and the consequences made clear, and a written programme guide has been discussed and given out;
4 to obtain, in the case of minors, the consent of parent or guardian;
5 to inform clients of the limits with regard to confidentiality;
6 to ensure that clients in group settings sign a document agreeing to maintain the confidentiality of group discussions.

This framework seems to be a useful start, as it applies general principles to the field of sex offender treatment. It should not be seen, either, as necessarily in conflict with Ross's statements, but as an ethical underpinning to the non-traditional approach he advocates.

With regard to confidentiality, Goring and Ward (1990) have usefully reviewed the legal position in the UK of practitioners working with sex offenders. Recognising that sex offenders may disclose further information about prior or even current offences, both before and after court hearings, they offer the following advice:

1 the legal advantages of offering express confidentiality are marginal;
2 any confidentiality is implicit and limited, because the public interest in disclosure would be likely to override the legal doctrine of confidentiality;
3 because of the above, the attendance of clients in treatment pre-sentence is often incompatible with the their legal interests, and should only take place with the agreement of their legal advisors;
4 a code of practice should be established covering the disclosure of information by treatment providers;
5 those working with offenders need to be aware that information supplied to other statutory agencies may be the basis of coercive intervention by such agencies;
6 given the above possibility, practitioners need to anticipate whether the

methods by which the information was obtained, for instance through group confrontation, are likely to withstand judicial scrutiny.

Tensions remain between practitioners from different disciplines about the exchange of sensitive information, which can interfere with collaboration. There is therefore a need for a code of practice, agreed preferably on an interagency basis. The intention here, however, is to provoke consideration of the issues, rather than to be prescriptive. The process of such discussion will in itself lead to a sharing of values, philosophies and theoretical understandings, and it is this that will lead to the best practice.

CONCLUSION

Working with sex offenders is a challenging field. Despite the understandable fears and fantasies, many practitioners have found the work to be highly rewarding, because of its clear emphasis on change. It is perhaps because of their apprehensions that practitioners have sought to approach this work in such a disciplined manner, relating research and theory to practice and evaluation. Many have remarked on the potential value of their approaches with sex offenders to other clients.

This chapter has sought to put in context the work that is described in the rest of the book. The local context of each reader's practice will have different strengths and constraints, and all of us must work creatively with those factors that lie beyond our control. Despite these contextual difficulties, the fact remains that what practitioners have achieved in this growing field has been very considerable. It is largely their skills and efforts which have succeeded in getting this work firmly on the political and managerial agenda. The final message, therefore, of this chapter is to prepare properly, set realistic and specific expectations, work with at least one colleague, and above all, to believe in the relevance of previous knowledge and skills.

NOTE

1 For a detailed description of the law relating to sex offenders, the reader is referred to Cowburn and Wilson (1992) *Changing Men* on the Criminal Justice Act, or the NCH Report (1992) on matters relating to the Children Act.

3 Assessment of sex offenders

Richard Beckett

INTRODUCTION

Assessment is a continuous process without defined boundaries, extending from the point at which abuse is suspected or detected, throughout treatment and beyond as long-term follow-up takes place. At each stage new information is obtained and the preceding assessment is revised accordingly. An initial risk assessment needs to describe offenders' developmental histories, the duration of their sexual problems, their level and pattern of denial, motivation for treatment and a basic description of the main problem areas as detailed in the third section of this chapter. This enables recommendations for treatment to be made. It will usually require a minimum of three hours of direct interviewing, to which must be added time for information gathering, discussion with other relevant parties, analysis of questionnaires and report writing.

This chapter has three sections which are ordered to reflect the usual sequence of assessment. The first section addresses the overall purpose and characteristics of an effective assessment and the problems associated with offenders' self-reporting. The second section considers the planning and conduct of the initial interview, with particular emphasis on overcoming denial, and the purpose and structure of taking a detailed personal history. The final section describes the assessment of particular offender problems: cognitive distortions, victim empathy, sexual arousal and fantasy, and finally social skills and competence. As each of these are addressed, subsections are devoted to the different ways of gathering information by clinical interview, through direct observation, the setting of homework assignments and the use of questionnaires.

The assessment procedures described are applicable to clients in both community and residential settings and can be used almost without exception by practitioners of any professional discipline. However, since assessment is a skill that must be learnt and since some assessment approaches are particular to sex offenders, it is not assumed that practitioners can use them all without training, practice supervision and access to discussion with more experienced colleagues.

Whilst Chapter 7 deals specifically with adolescent sex offenders, the division between older adolescents and young adults is indistinct and somewhat arbitrary. Some 17 year olds can present with a range and severity of problems very similar to those of adult offenders. The assessment of both adults and adolescents can therefore be similar, in that both present with patterns of denial and distortions, varying degrees of sexual arousal to children, apparent lack of victim empathy and relationship problems. Where they differ is generally in the degree to which their problems are entrenched – for example, younger offenders tend to have a less extensive range of distorted beliefs about sex offending and less well established deviant sexual arousal. Moreover, when addressing the problems of younger abusers, assessment needs to be adjusted to take account of their different developmental status, generally lower level of abstract reasoning, ability to articulate thoughts and feelings and their relative lack of sexual knowledge and experience. These differences will need to be reflected in the style and approach to assessment.

PURPOSE OF ASSESSMENT

The request for offender assessment may arise in a variety of circumstances. When sexual abuse is disclosed or suspected, child protection agencies must arrive at a decision as to the risk a suspected abuser presents, not only to the victim, but to other potentially vulnerable children. The probation service will most commonly be involved at the point where recommendation must be made to the courts regarding sentence. Psychologists and psychiatrists may be asked to provide assessment and opinion on risk, treatability and recommendation for disposal. Assessments may also be requested by child protection case conferences or parole boards, so that future plans can be made. Although the agencies may vary in their primary roles, all share the overriding objective of protecting children, and it is with this objective in mind that assessment takes place. The overall purposes of assessment are threefold: to evaluate the risk of reoffending; to identify treatment priorities and targets; and to evaluate treatment outcome.

To evaluate risk of reoffending and the level of dangerousness presented by the offender

Recidivism studies indicate that over the shorter term (up to five years) untreated child sex offenders vary in their reconviction rate (see Chapter 1). Intra-familial abusers of girls have the lowest levels of reconviction, with rates ranging from 4 to 10 per cent (Gibbens *et al.*, 1978, 1981). Extra-familial abusers of girls have reconviction rates in the range 10 to 29 per cent, with extra-familial abusers of boys having the highest reported reconviction rate: 13 to 40 per cent (Furby *et al.*, 1989). However, there is considerable variation within each group of offenders and assessment of the individual needs to be undertaken in order to identify those individual characteristic and situational circumstances which may result in reoffending.

Dangerousness is a multi-dimensional concept which incorporates likelihood of reoffending and escalation of offending behaviour, level of remorse, motivation to change, and the degree of trauma a new offence would cause. Considerations of dangerousness are particularly relevant to decisions regarding custodial versus community disposal and treatment, and are also considered in Chapter 4.

To inform decisions regarding treatment priority and the nature, target and context of intervention

When treatment resources are limited, agencies may be concerned to target offenders who are assessed as being at a relatively high risk of shorter-term recidivism. Regardless of which offenders are targeted for intervention, assessment is required to define the treatment needs of the individual and to develop individual relapse prevention packages.

To evaluate treatment effectiveness and to develop and refine intervention strategies

Treatment programmes vary according to their content and delivery, organisational structure, therapist skill mix and type of offenders accepted. Since even apparently similar programmes appear to vary in their effectiveness (Marshall, Ward, *et al.* 1991), assessment of treatment outcome is essential if programmes are to evaluate their strengths and weaknesses.

Characteristics of effective assessment

There are a number of principles which should guide the practitioner in ensuring abusers are adequately assessed.

Clear theoretical models

To fully understand sexual assault, a multi-factorial model is needed which can explain the internal motivation of the offender together with disinhibiting factors, and describe how a child became or was made vulnerable to assault. Possibly the most useful is the Finkelhor four-factor model (Finkelhor, 1984), outlined in Chapter 1.

Men who sexually assault children are not a homogeneous group, but vary according to their personal histories and presenting characteristics. They present with varying degrees of denial, deviant sexual arousal, victim preference, social competence, intellectual ability and maturity, etc. Assessment must ensure that these individual characteristics are taken into account in order to determine appropriate interventions. Knight's child molester typology (1988) provides one way of systematically classifying different types of men who sexually abuse children. Details of how to use this approach are to be found in Knight *et al.* (1989).

Recognising problems with offender self-report

Regardless of the assessment format used: verbal self-report, psychometric testing or psychophysiological measures (e.g. penile plethysmograph – see below), all approaches suffer from problems of reliability. Self-report by sex offenders is problematic, for a number of reasons. They rarely present willingly for assessment, and at interview they are often defensive and distorting. They may fear a negative response from the interviewer and negative consequences from the court or child protection system if they disclose the full extent of their sexual deviancy. Furthermore, even when apparently motivated to provide accurate accounts of their behaviour, research has demonstrated that considerable discrepancy may exist between independently observed and self-reported behaviour (e.g. Segal and Marshall, 1985). Moreover, the quality of information obtained by interview is highly dependent upon the experience and skills of the interviewer. Their skill in creating a non-collusive working alliance which encourages disclosure, their ability to ask assumptive questions and their sensitivity to transference or counter-transference issues will all influence the quality of offender disclosure. Further problems in self-report information caused by unsystematic ways of gathering information can be avoided by the use of structured interview schedules which prompt interviewers into covering the main assessment areas.

Determining reliability of self-report

Since most assessment measures are reliant on verbal or written self-report measures, the quality and reliability of information divulged needs to be judged against the individual's general willingness to disclose. If the offender resists disclosing, omits, distorts or is inconsistent in the accounts of previous non-abusive behaviour (as documented in the reports of others), then the reliability of his offence-related disclosures is brought into question.

Three broad approaches may be used to assist in judging the reliability of offender self-report. The most important is to ensure that there is a good level of agreement between offender self-report and those of others. Secondly, personality scales which incorporate validity scales (Lanyon *et al.* 1991), or procedures for adjusting self-report for social desirability bias (Saunders, 1991) may be used to alert interviewers to individuals who attempt to fake good or bad, or who lack insight into their general feelings and motives. Thirdly, scales may be employed which enable comparison to be made between the offender and other offenders of a similar type. In addition to its clinical scales and personal history, the multiphasic sex inventory (MSI) (Nicholls and Molinder, 1984) contains seven validity scales, standardised on treated and untreated sex offenders as well as non-offending males. The validity scales scores enable interviewer to judge the probability that an offender is responding truthfully to the questionnaire.

Although the MSI cannot prove an offender is lying, it again alerts to the possibility that he may be doing so.

Multiple sources of information

No single assessment approach is invulnerable to problems of faking by the subject. Consequently the reliability and validity of assessment is most likely to be improved, though not assured, when assessments combine information gathered from offender self-report, psychometric tests and the reports and behavioural observations of others. To this end, the following section, devoted to the assessment of specific offender characteristics, attempts to provide strategies for the gathering of data from multiple sources, including interviews, formal testing, behavioural observations, homework assignments, and the reports of others.

Throughout the chapter, reference is also made to the use of treatment tasks as sources of further information to inform the assessment process at a later stage. Wherever assessments rely on single sources of information, the practitioner should be alert to the probable reduction in the reliability of the assessment and be cautious in making recommendations based upon it.

INITIAL CONSIDERATIONS

Building the professional network

Before the initial interview, it is important to contact the key professionals in the child protection and criminal justice networks. A framework for information exchange should be established and individual roles in the overall assessment of the offender, the victim and their family agreed. Without this negotiation and the building of professional network, distorted dynamics between agencies are more likely to occur – the agency assessing the offender becoming contaminated with suspicion that they are sympathetic and collusive with the offender, the child protection agency being perceived within the assessment system as precipitate in their actions, unwilling to understand offender motives and denying the possibility of change. These and other dynamics, which in intra-familial abuse may mirror splits within the family system, create the danger of hostility and mistrust between professionals, and may result in poor quality, disjointed or conflicting recommendations being made to courts and child protection case conferences.

The victim's statement, case conference minutes, previous pre-sentence reports and the offender's previous convictions are also gathered at this stage, though the latter must be viewed cautiously since they may not be complete and their content may be misleading, as discussed in Chapter 1. The victim's statement is essential to the assessment, since without it no judgement of offender denial or admittance can be made. The victim's statement will contain details of assault behaviour, degree and nature of coercion, how the child was made vulnerable, the degree of immediate trauma suffered by the victim, and the situational circumstances surrounding the abuse. This information is also essential later in treatment for the detailed examination of the offender's thoughts and feeling and the identification of factors that may lead to future offending.

The time available for an initial assessment is often very limited, due to pressure from criminal courts or child protection agencies. Where reasonable time has not been allowed, written reports should record this and detail the assessment areas not adequately covered.

Denial and defence

Offenders may present at any point along a continuous line, from total denial through partial admittance with attendant minimisation and distortion, through to complete admittance. As Salter (1988) has observed, denial has a number of components. Offenders may admit abuse, but deny prior planning or deviant fantasy. They may admit to sexual contact with a child but deny that harm has occurred, or may portray the child as an active and willing participant in the abuse. Not uncommonly, offenders initially deny previous histories of assaults and sexually deviant behaviour, despite clinical experience and research studies (Abel *et al.*, 1987) which indicate the contrary.

Religious conversion or emotionality may also be used as a defence against assessment. Having 'found God', religious converts may attempt to persuade the practitioner that all future risks are now removed; that risk assessment is redundant. Other offenders may become highly distressed at interview, implicitly appealing to the sympathetic side of the helping and caring professional. Yet others may admit to all the accusations, in the hope that the interviewer will equate admission of guilt as synonymous with removal of future risk. The goal of treatment is to move beyond full admittance, to a point where the offender acknowledges the risk of future relapse and can demonstrate the behavioural, attitudinal and emotional changes which reduce relapse risk.

Motivational interview strategies

Whereas denial of previous sexual deviancy, of fantasy and planning may be tolerated during the early stage of assessment, outright denial of abuse or resistance to cooperate severely restricts the opportunity for meaningful assessment. Directly confronting the offender with the victim's account of their abuse may be successful in securing an admission. However, should this strategy fail it is difficult to retrieve the situation once outright denial in the face of confrontation has taken place. For this reason, motivational interviewing approaches may be used which anticipate offender resistance, maximise offender cooperation and establish a non-collusive, collaborative relationship within which later direct and sustained confrontation can take place if required.

Underpinning this approach is the assumption that denial, minimisation and other psychological defences have been constructed by the offender during the course of the abuse to help minimise his guilt and anxiety. Consequently interview approaches which intensify anxiety may strengthen defence and resistance, whereas strategies which moderate fear and anxiety may lessen the need for such defences and increase the likelihood of engaging the offender in a constructive dialogue. The following strategies are recommended to assist in reducing denial:

1 Explain the purpose of the assessment, its likely duration, what information will be sought, other professionals involved in the investigation and what information the interviewer has already gathered.

2 Acknowledge that the offence with which he is charged, and the accusations made, represent a life crisis for the client, insofar as he faces separation from his family, possible prosecution and imprisonment, loss of employment and publicity.

3 Present as confident and familiar with the dilemmas the offender faces in fully admitting to the extent of his sexual deviancy and the consequences of doing so.

4 Convey that in the interviewer's experience, whilst offenders feel anxious about fully disclosing and cooperating, many feel relief having done so, and are subsequently able to change and rebuild their lives, albeit and necessarily in a way different from before.

5 Explain the benefits of collaborating in the assessment, how it will create the opportunity for treatment and how cooperation will enable constructive recommendations to be made to the courts and child protection agencies. By contrast, denial will severely limit the range of recommendations that can be made, and narrow the range of options likely to be considered by the courts and statutory agencies. At the same time, practitioners must not guarantee that the courts or agencies will necessarily follow whatever recommendations are made on the basis of the assessment.

6 Communicate that despite what others may have said about the offender, and the view many offenders have of themselves – that they suffer a basic characterological defect – the interviewer takes the view that it is the person's behaviour which is the problem, and not necessarily the individual's core self and personality.

7 Make clear that the interviewer will be straight-forward with the offender and discuss the outcome of the assessment and its recommendation, thus creating a climate of truthfulness.

8 Make clear that information divulged will not be confidential, but shared with other professionals in the child protection network.

Having made these explicit statements and created the attendant expectations, the interviewer can adopt other strategies designed to further minimise denial and enhance disclosure. Amongst McGraths' (1990) suggestions are:

1 Developing a 'yes set', whereby initial non-controversial questions are framed so as to ensure affirmative answers to non-collusive questions, thus creating a climate of cooperation which can serve to minimise resistance when more searching questions are asked.

2 Ignoring answers believed to be untruthful and reframing the question at a later point in the interview, thus not allowing the offender to engage in and become entrenched in denial.

3 Employing 'successive-approximation strategies', whereby basic information is first obtained and progressively more detail is sought as the interview progresses. This helps ensure that the offender is not faced at the outset with having to disclose highly detailed and anxiety-laden material, thus reducing the probability of denial because of the anxiety of disclosure.
4 Emphasising the collaborative nature of the assessment and the offender's own need to understand why he offended. In this way the offender is invited to share with the interviewer a mutual endeavour of determining why the assaults took place and how they can be avoided in the future.

Whilst it is essential to gather the offender's account of the abuse during the initial assessment, it is also important to do this at a point where he is motivated to disclose. Motivation is enhanced when the offender feels the interviewer has some interest in him as an individual and in the cause of his sexual problems, and expresses concern to ensure he gets the appropriate help.

Consequently while a broad description of the offence is gathered at the first meeting, it is usually best to leave detailed questioning about the assaults until sufficient rapport has been established and the offender feels more motivated to cooperate. It is recommended therefore that a personal history is taken before detailed offence-specific questions are asked.

FOCUSES OF ASSESSMENT

A personal history

The purpose of gathering personal history details at this stage is threefold. First, to gather details of the offender's developmental experiences, which may help to explain the cause of his sexual offending. Second, details of the offender's recent history will help to identify those contemporary factors which may have contributed to the current cycle of offending. Finally, by concentrating at this stage upon personal history, the interviewer develops an awareness of the offender's personality style, his ability to recount events, and his general willingness to disclose, and builds a rapport with the offender, thus establishing a relationship within which later de tailed and confrontational questions may be asked.

A full psychosocial evaluation may focus upon a potentially wide range of areas: the characteristics of the offender's family of origin, the quality of his parenting, his early life experiences, social, sexual and educational history, and his medical, psychiatric, marital, occupational and criminal history. The reader is referred to Groth (1979) for a description of a comprehensive clinical interview.

While no predictive studies have been undertaken to identify developmental experiences which predict sexual offending in adulthood, a number of retrospective studies have identified experiences more prevalent in the life histories of men who sexually assault children, as opposed to those who rape adult women. Whilst studies are not unanimous, rapists tend toward histories of more frequent physical abuse, with parental punishment characterised as harsh, frequent and inconsistent (Rada, 1978) and with fathers, where present, being aggressive, criminal and drunken (Langevin *et al.*, 1985). Perhaps not surprisingly, rapists show patterns of conduct disorder in childhood and delinquency in adolescence. By contrast, those who sexually assault children tend not to have childhood patterns of childhood conduct disorder; rather they have poor or distant relationships with parents, are socially isolated from peers (Araji and Finkelhor, 1986) and a significant number have been sexually abused themselves as children (Becket *et al.*, 1994). As adults, child sex abusers vary considerably in their presenting characteristics. While some intra-familial offenders may display patterns of drug or alcohol abuse, sexual dysfunction, low esteem, dominance/authoritarianism, this is not universally the case. Similarly, extra-familial abusers share no single set of developmental or presenting characteristics. While some are socially incompetent, lack social skills and may be passive, dependent and isolated, others are socially skilled, assertive and successful. The key areas for assessment of previous history include the following factors.

Family of origin

- Parental criminality, anti-social behaviour and evidence of alcohol and drug abuse and its consequences for the offender and his family.
- The presence and degree of parental marital disharmony, and whether this resulted in physical violence and to whom it was directed.

Childhood

- Whether the offender was physically abused, emotionally rejected or isolated within his family and the reasons for and consequences of this.
- If he was sexually abused, the identity of the abuser, the duration of the abuse and the emotional and behavioural consequences for him.
- Any evidence of childhood behavioural, or neurotic disorders and their cause, duration and consequences.

- Did these result in referral to professional agencies?
- How did the offender relate to other children whilst growing up?
- Did any children become especially emotionally salient because, for example, his relationships with parents was poor or disrupted?
- Did the offender have health problems which disrupted family or school life?

School

- To what extent was he isolated, rejected or in conflict with his peers, and the reasons for this.
- Did this result in the offender socialising with younger children, to reduce the isolation?
- Was the offender in conflict with his teachers, as evidenced by punishment, suspension or expulsion?
- Details of and reason for referral to child guidance, counselling or special schooling.
- Did he fail or have academic difficulties, truant (alone or with peers), or show evidence of impulsivity, aggression or delinquent behaviour outside of school?

Sexual history

- History of offender's own experience of sexual victimisation and its consequences, emotionally, behaviourally and socially.
- His sexual learning experiences, evidence of unusual sexual or non-peer sexual encounters and how such experiences were understood both at the time and retrospectively.
- The extent to which earlier sexual encounters were the focus of sexual fantasy and masturbation and whether they continue to feature in current sexual fantasy.
- Exposure to, and use of pornography, its range and whether its use is habitual.
- His sexual orientation: when did this orientation become established, what relationships and sexual experiences contributed to this preference and did his sexual orientation result in difficulties or interpersonal conflicts whilst growing up?
- His history of sexual encounters, the degree to which partners have been age-appropriate, whether he has behaved coercively in sexual relations and the extent to which he views himself as socially and sexually competent with desired partners.

- His ability to establish and maintain intimate relationships, his level of sexual satisfaction in them, whether he has had sexual affairs outside of his main relationship or visited prostitutes.
- Where relationships have broken up, the reasons for this.

Occupational/social/recreational history

- The extent to which the offender has been successful in establishing himself in adult relationships, both social, intimate and economic, and his degree of satisfaction with them.
- Where employment has been available, failure to enter employment, or loss of employment may be indicative of conflict with work colleagues or employers and should be explored for evidence of social incompetency, or anxiety, alcohol abuse or anti-social behaviour.
- Whether the offender is or has been a member of social organisations, particularly where these may give access to social contact with children or whether he has recreation which involve child-centred activities.

Offending history

- Previous non-sexual offences should be considered in regard to their nature: offences against the person, against property, or social rule violations, e.g. drink/drive, their frequency, circumstances and motivation.
- When previous sexual offences are reported they identify the offender as more likely to be entrenched in his sexual deviancy and such previous offences will themselves become the focus of assessment.
- Details of the circumstances, motivation of these previous offences, and the characteristics of the victims, particularly in regard to whether the offender shows a pattern of escalation over time, whether previous offences suggest a preferred sex or victim type or show a pattern of cross-over between intra- and extra-familial abuse.

Contemporary events

The second main focus of personal history-taking is to identify those contemporary events and internal psychological processes which have contributed to precipitating the current period of sexual offending. Through this analysis, 'high-risk' elements can be identified and subsequently targeted for treatment.

Negative emotional states, interpersonal conflicts and social pressure are the immediate precursors of many relapses in individuals with addictive or compulsive behaviour (Cummings *et al.*, 1980). This also applies to sex offenders (Pithers *et al.*, 1988). In some cases life events, financial problems, loss of employment, bereavement or divorce, may be identified as causing a reduction in self-esteem, increasing loneliness or intensifying feelings of worthlessness, and thus creating the negative mood state which precedes the decision to offend. It should be noted, however, that not all abuse is preceded by negative emotional states in the offender. Some offenders harbour constant and high levels of deviant fantasy and arousal, cognitive distortion and motivation to abuse. In such cases the occurrence of offences is determined as much by availability of victims as by negative psychological states. In many cases, however, such specific and easily identifiable events will not be in evidence. Consequently the chain of external events, their impact on psychological processes and relationship to abuse onset may require extended exploration. This is a treatment task (see Chapter 4), but may be started during initial assessment by setting the offender an autobiographical assignment.

Throughout the assessment the interviewer needs to cross-check self-report wherever possible against the reports of others, such as the victims of his offences, family, partners, social services and, where appropriate, other agencies, e.g. previous employers.

Cognitive distortions

Distortion of attitude and belief, whereby children are portrayed as being in some way responsible for their own abuse, and that they are not harmed by sexual contact with adults and are able to consent to or gain benefit from such encounters is one of the most common characteristics exhibited by child sexual abusers (Abel, Becker, Cunningham-Rathner, *et al.*, 1984).

The identification of such distortions helps determine judgements of future risk, informs decisions regarding involvement of offenders in victims' therapy and reintegration of offenders back into their families. Offenders who remain convinced that some children are not harmed by sexual contact with adults, or that they actively seek such contact, will remain at risk of repeating their offending. If offenders have contact with their victims, for example in the context of offering an apology, whilst continuing to believe that the child secretly enjoyed the abuse, the victim will also remain vulnerable to psychological and emotional revictimisation.

Whilst for some offenders their cognitive distortion appears mainly associated with their current victim, others display distortions which are long-standing and pervasive. Such pervasive distortion may be the product of developmental experiences which have set the framework for distorted beliefs regarding children and sexuality in adulthood. For example, sexual encounters with peers whilst growing up may be subsequently construed as indicative of children's potential not merely to be sexually interested in peers but also in adults. Witnessing or suspecting sexual assaults by adults or by other children may inculcate beliefs that such behaviour is acceptable, and that children are legitimate targets of adult sexual interest. Men who have been sexually abused as children may feel responsible for precipitating their own abuse or colluding with it by failing to complain or resist. This may instil the belief that the abusing adult is not entirely responsible, that children can lead adults astray and choose not to disclose, because they secretly enjoy such experiences. Where offenders have abused before and not been adequately confronted or punished, their capacity to minimise or deny the victim's trauma may be reinforced by the response of those around them. Where harm has occurred, the offender may attribute this to child protection investigations or interventions, rather than the abuse itself.

Assessment

Some cognitive distortions appear relatively superficial and defend the offender against feelings of anxiety and guilt. Such defence mechanisms include denial, repression, minimisation and externalising blame onto life stresses, marital problems or alcohol.

Other distortions, however, may be deeply held. For example, a statement to the effect that 'some children want sexual contact with adults' may be a superficial justification, or a deeply held and entrenched belief. Offenders with a fixated sexual interest in children typically display a range of more fundamental distortions, related to the belief that some children will actively seek sexual encounters with adults, can consent to and benefit from such encounters and have the capacity to reciprocate the degree of emotional feeling and attachment the adult abuser may feel for the child. One of the assessment tasks is to separate superficial distortions of defence from those which are more deeply entrenched, since the latter are commonly associated with a sexual preference for children and indicate an individual at greater risk of reoffending. The goal of assessment is therefore to elicit specific details of each distortion, the perceived attributes, characteristics and behaviour of children which trigger such distortions, whether certain moods or situations make such distortions more likely to occur, and how offenders behave when such distortions occur.

Clinical interview

Distortions of attitude and belief commonly emerge when the offender is asked to provide a detailed account of his offending behaviour and this is compared with the victim's report. Where the offender portrays the child as sexually provocative, that s/he enjoyed or was not harmed by the abuse, the interviewer may feel impelled to immediately challenge such statements. The purpose at this stage is, however, to elicit as many such statements as possible which are indicative of cognitive distortions.

While not colluding with the offender, the interviewer needs to encourage the expression of as many hidden beliefs as possible and to record their content. If confrontation occurs too early, offenders will acquiesce, and their beliefs will remain undisclosed and, therefore, not amenable to assessment. Disclosure is facilitated when the interviewer uses an enquiring tone, and offers hypotheses as to what the offender might have thought regarding a child's behaviour towards him. For example:

Interviewer:	'You've told me that on several occasions before you assaulted your daughter [age 12 years] that you had complained to your wife about her walking around downstairs with only her nightie on. You had also noticed that she was developing breasts. What do you think was going through her mind when she did this?'
Offender:	'She was just trying it on, trying to wind me up.'
Interviewer (hypothesises):	'Perhaps you thought she was being deliberately sexually provocative?'
Offender:	'Dead right, she knew exactly what she was doing, she was a little madam, hanging around with all those boys, flaunting herself, she was turning into a slut.'

By offering the above hypothesis, but not colluding with it, the interviewer elicits themes of bed-time behaviour misattributed as sexually motivated, misrepresentation of normal adolescent peer group behaviour (being with boys, perhaps a developing sexual awareness), and denigration of her into a sexual object (slut), used together as a rationalisation for his sexual assaults.

Specific questions can also be put which invite disclosure of further distortion, for example:

Interviewer:	'Thinking about the way the child behaved towards you, what did he do or say which led you to believe he did not mind or was interested in having sexual contact with you?'

More deeply held distortions may also emerge during treatment as the offender becomes more open and actively engaged in examining the details of his offending behaviour. As his planning of assaults is admitted and his pattern of grooming victims is exposed, his rationale for selecting one victim as opposed to another will become clearer, as will those characteristics of children which provoke distortions and strong feelings within the offender.

Emotional congruence

For some fixated offenders in particular, cognitive distortions may also be accompanied by distorted emotional attachments to children. For such offenders children fulfil emotional as well as sexual needs, and frequently such men have corresponding difficulties in making and sustaining adult relationships (Beckett *et al.*, 1994). These men make statements indicating an emotional over-responsiveness, identification and dependence upon children. The origin of this emotional congruence can usually be traced back to special emotional or sexual relationships with other children during the offender's own childhood or early adolescence. Statements indicating high emotional congruence include: 'Children seem to seek me out', 'Children remind me of myself', 'Children stop me feeling lonely', 'I am better than most people at getting along with children'.

Assessment

Whether as part of the assessment or in the content of treatment, offenders' responses to therapeutic exercises and material also provides an important means of assessing cognitive distortions. Their response to video tapes of survivors talking, particularly when they are asked to compare and contrast these with their own victims' experience, typically elicits defensiveness and distortions. Similarly their response to therapeutic reading material and their victim apology letters (see Chapter 4) will also often reveal distortions.

Homework assignments may require offenders to bring back examples of published and broadcast material which 'triggers' or confirms their underlying suspicion regarding, for example, children's sexual intention towards adults. Offenders may also be asked to keep a diary or report verbally upon children's behaviour which might potentially put the child at risk, and these examples can be used as a framework within which to consider the cognitive distortions involved. Distortions may also be assessed indirectly by analysing masturbatory satiation audio tapes (see Chapter 4). As a by-product of this treatment, offenders' deviant fantasies can be analysed for statements and descriptions of victim's behaviour, e.g.: victim seducing the offender or enjoying the encounter, which distort the actual reality of sexual assaults and impact on victims. Finally 'victim apology letters', written as a victim empathy treatment task, may also provide additional examples of distortion which can be the subsequent focus of treatment intervention (see Chapter 4).

Questionnaire approaches

The Abel and Becker cognition scale (Abel and Becker, 1984) and the justifications (Ju) and cognitive distortion and immaturity scales (CDI) of the MSI (Nichols and Molinder, 1984) are the most widely available scales for assessing cognitive distortions. The Abel and Becker scale contains statements concerning adult sexual contact with children, and respondents are asked to what extent they agree or disagree with each one. For example:

> 'Sex between a 13 year old (or younger) child and an adult causes the child no emotional problems.'
> 'Sometime in the future, our society will realise that sex between a child and an adult is all right.'

Unfortunately, while the Abel and Becker scale has high face validity there are few reports as to the reliability of the scale, and it suffers from being transparent and vulnerable to faking. Consequently when offenders do not endorse questionnaire items this should not be taken to mean that distortions do not exist.

Victim empathy

Empathy describes an individual's ability to accurately perceive and respond to the feelings of others. Several studies of child abusers have indicated they are impaired in their capacity for empathy, particularly towards their own victim (e.g. Beckett *et al.*, 1994). Developmental experiences, particularly lack of parental affection, harsh and non-contingent punishment, have been implicated in producing adults who are emotionally unresponsive and indifferent to the feelings of others. However, even for individuals who have developed the capacity for empathic responding, this may be suspended or overridden in certain circumstances. When victims are perceived as deserving of abuse, guilty of provoking or enjoying sexual contact with adults, their distress is likely to be ignored. It may be that without the development of such cognitive distortion, empathic feelings for the victim would inhibit such abuse occurring or decrease the likelihood of its escalation after an initial abusive encounter.

Certain mood states, particularly anger or sexual arousal, are also able to overcome empathic responding. Finally some offenders may show lack of empathy because in the absence of a victim's overt distress they may lack the basic knowledge as to the distress likely to be suffered by the victim and the serious longer-term consequences that can follow.

Clinical interview

In practice the assessment of victim empathy is often undertaken in the course of identifying and treating cognitive distortions, since it is only by their modification that the degree to which an offender can empathise can be fully determined. Evidence from other areas of the offender's life, their self-reported feelings and reports of those who have relationships with the offender, assist the interviewer in determining whether the lack of empathy he showed to his victim is but an example of his general inability to be emotionally responsive, or the opposite, and help provide a composite picture of the offender's ability to perceive and respond to the feelings of others.

Behavioural exercises

Empathy and emotional responsiveness may also be assessed by observing and asking offenders to report their reactions to reading material and video tapes presented, either individually or in groups, during assessment and treatment. Such exercises may draw upon selected material from books such as *Kiss Daddy Goodnight* (Armstrong 1978) or *Betrayal of Innocence* (Forward and Buck 1978), articles and tapes made by survivors of sexual abuse, and television documentaries. Offenders can then rate the distress and other effects suffered by the victim portrayed on simple scales, which can then be used as baseline measures for subsequent change. Writing 'victim apology' letters or accounts of their offences from the victim's perspective are also effective means of examining offenders' empathic abilities and can again be used as baselines against which future change can be measured. In these exercises cognitive distortions frequently emerge and will need to be resolved before empathic responding is improved.

Questionnaires

Empathy is considered to have two distinct components:

1 cognitive role-taking ability, in which a person can imagine and accurately perceive others' thoughts and feelings;
2 emotional responsiveness, which describes the observer's capability to emotionally respond to such perceptions.

Of the most widely used empathy scales, the Mehrabian and Epstein Empathy Scale (1972) contains questions related only to empathic emotional responsiveness, whereas the Interpersonal Reactivity Scale (Davis, 1980) contains items related to cognitive role-taking and emotional responsiveness. Surprisingly, despite the emphasis given to developing victim empathy there are no reports to date of the use of these scales with men who sexually assault children.

Sexual arousal and fantasy

Psychophysiological measures of sexual arousal

Despite its clinical and research value as a means of directly assessing sexual preference, the penile plethysmograph (PPG) has not been widely adopted in the UK. While this is a specialist laboratory-based assessment procedure, it is important that practitioners are aware of its clinical and research value, even though they may not have access to one.

The device consists of a strain gauge, usually a thin metal band or mercury in a rubber loop, which when placed around the subject's penis measures change in size or, more specifically, tumescence.

The assessment procedure involves presenting the offender with visual slides depicting males and females of various ages, ranging from young children through to mature adults, and recording the offender's sexual response to them. The visual stimuli can be combined with the presentation of audio-taped recordings which portray varying degrees of coercion, from explicit aggression and forced sex through implicit threat, and in the case of children, seduction by manipulated consent. The offender's sexual response is then compared to his reaction to consenting sex between adults. Although the penile plethysmograph can be vulnerable to faking, and its results require skilled interpretation (Simon and Schouter, 1992), it remains the most reliable and valid means of assessing sexual preference, and has been particularly valuable in differentiating the sexual preferences of child sexual abusers.

A variety of studies have consistently demonstrated that many extra-familial abusers have sexual preferences for children (Freund, 1987; Quinsey, Chaplin and Carrigan, 1979). Studies of intra-familial abusers have varied in their findings, some studies finding them to have deviant sexual preferences similar to extra-familial child abusers (Abel *et al.*, 1981; Murphy *et al.*, 1986), while the studies of Freund and Quinsey found intra-familial abusers to have sexual preferences similar to non-offenders. Barbaree and Marshall (1989) found that with both intra- and extra-familial child sexual abusers against girls, five distinct patterns of sexual preference could be identified, thus indicating the existence within both types of offender of a considerable diversity of sexual preference. It is possible that a similar variety of response patterns will also be found with extra-familial abusers of boys.

Whilst the plethysmograph, in common with other assessment procedures, cannot prove the guilt of a non-admitting offender, even where a clearly deviant arousal pattern is found, it can be effective in helping challenge those offenders who deny their guilt. Marshall and Eccles (1991) have, for example, found that some of the men referred to their out-patient clinic who initially claimed innocence, subsequently admitted their guilt when confronted with the results of the plethysmograph assessment. Unfortunately since the plethysmograph is not available to many practitioners, alternative means of assessing sexual preference must be employed. One approach is to employ the Abel and Becker Sexual Interest Card Sort (Abel and Becker 1985), the other is the assessment of deviant sexual fantasy.

Sexual fantasy

Where direct psychophysiological measures of sexual arousal are not available, sexual fantasy can also provide a guide to sexual preference. Offenders vary in the extent to which they report sexual fantasies about children or adolescents. Fixated child abusers typically report child-focused sexual arousal and fantasies which may be of many years standing, often developing during adolescence or early adulthood. By contrast, non-fixated child abusers typically report a preponderance of sexual fantasies focused upon adult partners, with any child-focused fantasies normally focused on their current sexual victim. Since deviant sexual fantasy appears closely associated with deviant arousal, the assessment of fantasy provides an important means of establishing the degree to which an offender is fixated on children. Where deviant fantasy is pervasive and long-standing, it is indicative of fixated sexual interest and this knowledge informs judgement regarding the increased risk of further offending. Irrespective of the degree of fixed sexual preference, many offenders report sexual fantasies focused upon the victim they have abused. If not in the period leading up to the initial assault, once they have begun a series of sexual assaults, offenders frequently report having sexual fantasies focused upon the victim they are abusing. Wolf (1984) suggests that these recurrent deviant fantasies serve to overwhelm whatever feelings of transitory guilt the offender may experience immediately following an assault and contribute to disinhibiting the next assault. In this regard deviant fantasy is considered one of the central components in maintaining abusive behaviour.

Clinical interview

The assessment goal is to determine the content of deviant fantasies, their duration, frequency, the range of external stimuli, and internal states which trigger or intensify them and how they find behavioural expression. The private nature of sexual fantasies, combined with the fear that censure will take place if deviant fantasies are disclosed, makes their assessment problematic. Moreover, some offenders may not be engaging in deviant fantasies during the period of initial assessment. Consequently their full extent cannot always be determined early in the assessment process, and it may take a period of treatment before they are adequately described. Success in eliciting deviant fantasies is increased if the interviewer is comfortable with the use of sexually explicit language, demonstrates a familiarity with the range and substance of such fantasies, and is knowledgeable about the relationship between arousal, fantasy and behaviour. In addition, a range of working assumptions should guide the interviewer in assessing sexual fantasy:

1   sexual fantasies are a guide to sexual arousal;
2   sexual fantasies are constructed from memories attached to previous sexual experiences and also represent desired outcomes of future sexual encounters;
3   the more long-standing the deviant sexual fantasy, the greater is the probability that it will find behavioural expression;
4   sexual fantasies are strengthened by masturbation;
5   deviant fantasies may be more prevalent and accessible to assessment when self-esteem is low or threatened;
6   deviant and non-deviant sexual fantasies may coexist. Thus during masturbation an individual may move from non-deviant to deviant fantasies in order to sustain sexual arousal;
7   the relationship between deviant sexual fantasy and the behavioural expression of sexual deviancy is complex. While the presence of deviant fantasies increases the probability of sexual deviancy, it does not guarantee it.

Based on the assumption that deviant fantasies have or are currently occurring, interviewers can phrase their questions accordingly, for example:

'Out of ten occasions when you masturbate, on how many occasions do you find yourself thinking about the child you assaulted/children you find attractive/ etc?'
'I recall from our discussion of your adolescent sexual experiences that you had [for example] witnessed a friend sexually touching a child – how often do you find yourself thinking back to this and getting sexually aroused?'

'Since you have received no treatment as yet, I am expecting that you continue to have sexual fantasies about the child you have assaulted. Let's talk about them.'

'Many men find that certain moods make fantasies about children more likely to occur. What moods make your fantasies more frequent or intense?'

Homework assignment

Homework assignments set between assessment or therapy sessions are valuable in enabling the offender to record sexual thoughts, feelings and fantasies at, or close to, the time they actually occur. This improves the quality of detail and provides a more accurate guide to both their frequency and those events and mood states which trigger or intensify such fantasies. In practice, such assignments require considerable offender motivation, and sufficient compliance may not be achieved until after the initial assessment and when the offender is actively engaged in treatment. For offenders who report currently masturbating to deviant fantasy, their content may be sampled by asking the individual to write down or verbalise his current fantasies whilst masturbating and to record his fantasies directly onto audio tape. Before embarking upon this procedure, clear instructions are given that the focus of sampling is existing fantasies. However, to avoid strengthening such fantasies it is essential that this is exercise is set within a treatment context and arrangements made for active treatment, through covert sensitisation or masturbatory satiation training soon after the assessment exercise is complete (see Chapter 4).

Questionnaires

The Wilson Sexual Fantasy Questionnaire (Wilson, 1978) and the deviant fantasy subscales of the MSI are the most commonly available fantasy questionnaires. Again such questionnaires are vulnerable to offender denial and the effect of social desirability. Consequently, whilst assessment is enhanced if offenders endorse items on such questionnaires, if they fail to do so it does not mean that such fantasies are absent. Such questionnaire results must be interpreted cautiously and preferably in conjunction with measures of offender denial. In this respect the MSI which has been standardised on untreated and treated sex offenders, and which contains additional scales enabling judgements of denial to be made, has distinct advantages over the Wilson fantasy checklist.

Social skills and competence

Interpersonal skill deficits and social anxiety have long been implicated as factors contributing to the development and maintenance of sexually assaultive behaviour. Competent social behaviour requires skills in accurately perceiving and interpreting the social behaviour of others, an ability to generate and select the most socially appropriate response and the behavioural skills to carry out the behaviour (McFall, 1990). Men who sexually assault children have been found to have problems with assertion (Beckett *et al.*, 1994), poor social problem-solving skills (Barbaree *et al.*, 1988b), a fear of being negatively evaluated by others (Overholsen and Beck, 1986), histories of intimacy failure and emotional loneliness (Garlick, 1991) and social skill deficits (Segal and Marshall, 1985) and are reported as having problems in relating to other adults, especially women.

Issues at interview

Except in extreme cases where behavioural skill deficits or social anxiety are manifestly obvious, the assessment of an offender's social competence by interview alone is problematic. Not only are significant components affecting social performance hidden, e.g. fear of being negatively evaluated, but competence varies across situations. Consequently a social skill problem such as poor eye contact, unassertive style, difficulty in self-expression, which is evident at interview may simply be a response to the interview situation, and not representative of the offender's behaviour in general. Conversely an apparently competent social performance at interview, particularly where the interviewer structures the interaction, may be a poor guide to the offender's competence in less structured, informal situations, or those which require friendship-making skills or the ability to manage conflict. Account must also be taken of the interviewer's gender, their status and their own social competence in influencing the social behaviour of the offender at interview. Finally, when questioning the offender about his social competency, the interviewer must be aware that self-report does not necessarily correspond with behaviour, as observed in actual social interactions (Segal and Marshall, 1985).

The offender's interview behaviour and self-reported difficulties in social relationships are nevertheless important in identifying areas for more structured examination. Consequently, when offenders display anxiety or apparent skill deficits at interview, they need to be asked directly whether this is typical of them, or particular to the interview situation.

The offender's educational and employment histories, his pattern of friendships, dating and membership of social organisations, all provide a guide to his social competence. Particular attention should be paid to his ability to initiate and maintain intimate relationships. Where avoidance of them has occurred, or they have failed, the reasons for this need to be carefully examined, not only for evidence of skill deficits but also with regard to his underlying beliefs, attitudes and expectation. The offender's ability to manage interpersonal conflict, whether he habitually resorts to avoidance, submission or aggression as opposed to appropriate assertion and his pattern of blame attribution also need to be assessed.

Behavioural observations

Direct observation of the offender's social behaviour, supplemented by interviews and questionnaires and the reports of others, provides the most valid means of assessing social competence. Observation of offenders in therapeutic groups is valuable but the social situation is unrepresentative of normal situations. When offenders are placed in hostels this provides a particularly valuable setting in which to assess social problems, for instance a tendency towards social isolation, frequency of conflict and conflict resolution skills.

Role play provides the most practical means of assessing social skills. Not only can a wide variety of social situations be explored, but it is a format within which cognitive processes, problem solving, attribution and perceived self efficacy can also be explored. Standard role plays, when video recorded, can provide a baseline against which to measure therapeutic change.

Homework

Structured assignments may be set between sessions with offenders asked to report on their social difficulties and the circumstances in which these occur. Questionnaires or structured recording forms may be drawn up to assist the client in reporting their social anxiety, cognitions and behaviour and the behaviour of others towards them.

Questionnaires

There is a wide variety of questionnaires available which measure various elements of social skills and assertions (see Hollin and Trower, 1986), as well as aggression (see Goldstein and Keller, 1987), and which can be used both diagnostically and as measures for change. Relatively few, however, have been used systematically with sexual offenders against children.

Those which have include the Fear of Negative Evaluation Scale (Watson and Friend, 1969), and the Subjective Anxiety and Distress Scale (ibid).

CONCLUSION

Combining information derived from an assessment with knowledge as to the known characteristics of recidivist sex offenders provides the basis upon which to judge the immediate and longer-term risk an offender may present, his treatability and the priority treatment tasks.

Regardless of whether practitioners have access to formal psychological tests and measures, this chapter illustrates that much can be achieved through skilful clinical interviews. This is particularly the case where these are combined with therapeutic tasks designed to elicit the underlying thoughts and feelings of abusers. However, where standardised tests are not used, it is particularly important for practitioners to adopt a structured and systematic approach to assessment, since this creates the opportunity for periodically retesting clients during treatment. In some areas, for example personal history-taking, structured interview formats are relatively easy to design. In other areas, for example monitoring the frequency and focus of deviant sexual fantasies, practitioners will be faced with having to develop their own scales to assist monitoring change that takes place during treatment. It is through the development and use of such measures of change that the best quality decisions can be made as to when a client is ready to be discharged from treatment into maintenance programmes.

4 Cognitive-behavioural treatment of sex offenders

Richard Beckett

INTRODUCTION

This chapter reviews the most commonly used treatment approach in the UK with men who sexually assault children: cognitive-behavioural interventions. These interventions focus on altering patterns of deviant arousal, correcting distorted thinking, and increasing social competence, with educational input assisting offenders to gain knowledge in sexual matters, the effects of sexual abuse and sexual assault cycles.

Starting with a consideration of the components of current comprehensive treatment programmes, the first section covers general treatment issues, the treatability of offenders and the decision to offer community-based treatment. The next section considers the nature of the treatment contract, and the selection of treatment goals. The remainder of the chapter describes the sequence of therapy and the treatment of the main problems presented by offenders, and how therapeutic change can be measured and treatment gains maintained.

COMPREHENSIVE TREATMENT

Although some authors have raised questions regarding the overall efficiency of sex offender treatment programmes (Furby *et al.*, 1989), several recent outcome studies, reviewed by Marshall, Ward *et al.* (1991), give cause for cautious optimism. Whilst no treatment approach is 100 per cent effective for all offenders all of the time, certain offenders do appear to benefit from particular types of intervention, as indicated by reduced recidivism. In considering the components of most effective sex offender treatment programmes, it is noteworthy that there is no evidence to support the use of traditional analytic, insight-oriented or self-help approaches with these offenders. The majority of specialised programmes combine individual and group approaches utilising educational, cognitive-behavioural and family system intervention strategies (Knopp and Stevenson, 1988). With intra-familial offenders in particular, family therapy is a critical component if successful rehabilitation is to be attempted (see Chapter 8). As treatment programmes have developed, increasing emphasis is now being placed on incorporating relapse prevention strategies (e.g. Pithers and Cumming, 1989) as a means of maintaining treatment gains.

Given that offenders come into treatment with a mixture of problems, it is understandable that the trend is towards comprehensive treatment packages. It is not clear, however, what combination of interventions are necessary to reduce reoffending, and whether some are more critical to long-term therapeutic success than others. It is conceivable that for some offenders, removal of cognitive distortions, improved ability to recognise and avoid risk-taking behaviour and improved interpersonal skills might be sufficient, even though they continue to have deviant arousal patterns. For this reason, whilst we strive to be as comprehensive as possible, we should not be deterred from treating these offenders if we cannot meet all their needs. Rather, we need to evaluate our interventions and try to select those clients who appear, on the basis of longer-term follow-up, to benefit most from the particular combination of skills and interventions we can offer.

General treatment issues

Whilst the majority of interventions described in this chapter can be applied in either individual or group treatment contexts, some are more easily provided individually, as this allows time for detailed behavioural analysis, individually tailored intervention and review (e.g. covert sensitisation, described below). Other interventions, such as victim empathy training, appear especially effective when used in group settings where discussion and feedback from other offenders assists the therapeutic process, as described in Chapters 5, 6 and 7. Ideally, treatment programmes should be resourced to offer combinations of both individual and group approaches, so that the full range of offender needs can be met.

In reviewing the main components of cognitive-behavioural treatment, it is not intended to provide a detailed guide to their use and further reading will be necessary to gain knowledge in these treatment approaches. In principle, however, with further reading and supervised practice, all of the approaches described can be used by professionals of any relevant discipline, although with some treatment techniques, like covert sensitisation and masturbatory satiation, specific training and supervised practice will be required before use with patients or clients. Managers have a responsibility to ensure that practitioners have access to the training and supervision required.

Although this chapter describes cognitive-behavioural interventions, it is important in using these approaches that practitioners draw on all their usual counselling and therapeutic skills to help engage an offender in treatment.

All the treatment approaches described can be used with both adults and, with careful selection, older adolescent offenders. With the latter, treatment will need to be adjusted to take account of their stage of development, lower level of abstract reasoning and more concrete thinking styles by, for example, more use of practical exercises. Additionally, when offering treatment to adolescents it is important to ensure that they, and their carers are fully informed about, and in agreement with, the treatment programme.

The amount of time needed to treat an offender depends on a number of variables, including the severity of his problems, his motivation, therapist skills and treatment resources. Non-fixated offenders are generally in treatment for an average of 75 hours, whilst fixated offenders will usually require in excess of 150 hours of individual and group treatment before joining a maintenance programme, although this excludes time spent on homework assignments.

Finally, whilst focusing on work with individual offenders, whether or not this takes place in a group context, it is not intended that this work be seen in isolation from therapeutic work which may be taking place in parallel with victims and non-abusing partners. Indeed, with intra-familial offenders, it is essential that any consideration of family reunification is preceded by offender–partner, partner–victim, offender–victim and family work, which may include non-abused siblings, as discussed in Chapter 8.

Treatability

Decisions to offer treatment, the selection of treatment goals and recommendation regarding the most appropriate treatment setting and programme needs to be made on the basis of a systematic and comprehensive assessment, as described in Chapter 3.

McGrath (1991) identifies three basic conditions which must be met before an offender is considered ready for treatment: he must acknowledge that he has committed an offence and be prepared to accept some responsibility for it; he must perceive his offending as a problem – if not initially for his victim, at least for himself; and he must be willing to enter and actively participate in treatment. However, even when these basic criteria are fulfilled, decisions are still required as to whether, at what point, and under what circumstances, community-based treatment should be recommended.

Offenders who are mentally ill will require psychiatric treatment before a decision can be made as to whether the offending behaviour requires specific intervention. Whilst a small number of mentally ill people do sexually offend directly as a consequence of psychiatric disturbance, in many more cases the illness is secondary or unrelated to the offending, and requires intervention once the acute phase of the illness has been resolved. Where major drug or alcohol dependency exists, this will also need to be controlled before the sexual offending can be treated. This may require attendance at other specialised programmes before, or concurrently with, sex offence specific therapy.

For the majority of offenders, however, mental illness or serious substance abuse is not at issue. Learning difficulty in itself should not be a factor leading to exclusion from treatment, although such individuals may require a specialised treatment programme adjusted for their particular needs (see Chapters 3 and 6).

Recommending community treatment

Having determined whether or not an offender is basically amenable to treatment, a decision also needs to be made as to whether and under what conditions treatment in the community might be recommended. Leaving aside considerations related to societal demands for punishment, retribution and deterrence, the likelihood that an offender will reoffend early on during treatment, or not comply with restrictions placed upon him, are the major factors influencing the recommendation for community-based treatment. When abusers reoffend early on in treatment, not only have further children been victimised and society failed to be protected, but treatment programmes may also be jeopardised through loss of public and institutional confidence and support. Consequently caution should be exercised when considering recommending high-risk offenders for initial community-based treatment.

Unfortunately the prediction of recidivism is a complex and inexact science. While on the one hand the consequences of failing to identify a high-risk offender may be very serious, practitioners must also guard against a general tendency to over-predict violence and to over-estimate our clinical decision-making ability (Turk and Salovey, 1988). In fact, statistical methods of risk prediction are generally better than clinical ones (Sawyer, 1966).

Research has identified a number of developmental and presenting characteristics more prevalent in those men who are at higher risk of sexually offending against children. Such factors identified by McGrath (1991) and Thornton and Travers (1991) include a previous history of sexual or aggressive offences, multiple paraphilias, multiple victims, male and female victims or male victims only, extra- as opposed to intra-familial abuse, deviant sexual arousal, learning difficulty, few social supports and unstable employment history.

Ideally, these higher-risk offenders should be offered initial treatment in settings such as prison or specialist residential establishments. However, even with the development of prison service treatment programmes, many offenders will continue to return to the community presenting a relatively high risk of reoffending. In such circumstances parole restrictions on where offenders can live on release need to be sought and enforced as part of a package of external mandates which compel such individuals to enter and actively participate in treatment and maintenance programmes.

TREATMENT CONTRACTS

Treatment begins with the drawing up of a contract between the offender and therapist which specifies the terms, conditions and expectations under which treatment will take place. With intra-familial abusers, this contract needs to be written in collaboration with the relevant child protection agency. For incarcerated offenders it is agreed as part of their condition of parole. While the contracts are tailored to the requirements of individual offenders, they usually specify the frequency of treatment, the requirement for their active participation in therapeutic tasks, consequences of non-compliance with treatment, conditions of residence and parole, action to be taken if a child is suspected to be at risk, and a waiver of confidentiality.

Setting treatment goals

It is also at the stage of treatment contracting that a broad treatment plan and criteria-based treatment targets are set (see Table 4.1). In agreeing this, a balance needs to be struck between maximising the offender's participation in defining his treatment needs, whilst the therapist ensures that they remain in control and sets an agenda which covers all necessary treatment areas.

The treatment plan will not be comprehensive at this stage, as not all problems can be identified and sufficiently described until treatment has begun. This should be recognised by both client and therapist, and further treatment planning or review meetings set. Such new problem areas may then be added to the therapeutic contract or entered into the client's work book which, as it grows, can form the basis of his personal relapse prevention manual.

Initial assessment identifies a range of offender problems which are potential targets for treatment. Assuming change takes place as a result of

therapeutic intervention, at what
lem has been sufficiently resolv
itself be an inadequate guide to
since problems resolve, if at all,
severity, offender motivation and an
quently, in setting treatment goals,
where possible, be specified in advan
whether these targets are met. For so
peutic success might specify that the pr
would be the case for masturbation to de
blames his victim for the offence. In oth
specify an increase in a behaviour or be
example, specifying that an offender mus̲.   ₒ̲ about
the effects of sexual abuse to an agreed le   .ᵥ ιo recognise and
challenge cognitive distortions effectivel̖. ιn other areas criteria for
success might be defined as the development of a new skill, for example the
ability to specify those thoughts, feelings and behaviours which would
combine together to constitute a high risk of relapse. Other targets might
specify that offenders complete homework assignments, or reach a point
where they are able to describe to significant others, behaviour which
might indicate they were at risk of reoffending. However, whilst such
progress is an important indicator in the short term, sustained changes in
thinking and behaviour over time will be needed to indicate longer-term
reduction of risk.

Agreeing explicit therapeutic targets promotes an open and honest dialogue between the offender and therapist, helps ensure informed consent,
and reduces measuring change by time served in treatment. Table 4.1
illustrates a range of goals that could be specified as treatment objectives.

86　Sexual offending against childr...

Table 4.1 Treatment objectives

Inte...

Focus

Motivation

SEQUENCE OF TREATMENT

Because, during treatment, emphasis is given to active participation in
therapeutic exercises between sessions, it is useful to introduce such tasks
as early as possible, thus creating appropriate expectations about the treatment to come. Where resistance to this is encountered, the therapist needs
to restate the conditions and expectations of treatment, to concentrate on
building motivation and to use whatever external mandates are available to
their maximum effect. Such initial tasks may include completing questionnaires, reading offence-relevant articles, keeping a self-report diary or
beginning to write a sexual autobiography.

With regard to the initial focus of treatment, continuing to build up a
detailed picture of the cognitive behavioural chain of offending is productive,

	...ventions (include)	*Desired outcomes*
	• use of external controls and mandates for treatment	• regular attendance for treatment
	• negative consequences for non-compliance	• active participation in treatment
	• developing a 'collaborative' approach with offender	• completion of homework assignments
	• explicit and agreed treatment goals	
	• respect for client	
Denial	• detailed analysis of offending behaviour	• increased congruence between offender's and victim's accounts of assaults
	• working through victims' statements	• acknowledgement of offence planning, victim harm, deviant fantasy, need for treatment, future risk
	• non-aggressive confrontation	• admission of undetected offences
Offending behaviour	• detailed analysis of cognitive-behavioural chain/cycle of offending	• able to specify high-risk situations and behaviours
	• analysis of 'apparently irrelevant decisions' (AIDs)	• knows own internal and external triggers of risk
	• training in problem solving, avoidance, escape and coping strategies	• demonstrates problem solving and coping
	• partner alert list	• stable mood and tolerance of frustration
		• partner agrees to monitor offender
		• accepts risk exists
Deviant sexual arousal and fantasies	• education about link between fantasy, arousal and offending	• removal of deviant arousal
	• satiation training	• increase in non-deviant arousal
	• covert sensitisation	• recognition that deviant fantasy in future will indicate risk of relapse

Table 4.1 Continued

Focus	Interventions (include)	Desired outcomes
Cognitive distortions	• education on link between distortions and offending • challenging denial and distortions • reattribution training • role-reversal exercises • examination of offender's own abuse • analysis of offender's deviant fantasies	• absence of distortions • recognition of children's characteristics which evoke distortions • recognition of role of distortions in relapse risk
Victim empathy	• removal of cognitive distortions • education on impact of sexual abuse • reviewing consequences of own abuse • role play • studying victim's account of their abuse • writing victim apology letters	• ability to describe consequences of sexual abuse • acknowledgement of damage done to own victim • correct victim apology letter
Interpersonal skills	• social skill, assertion and anger management training	• expressed satisfaction with increased social competence • reduction in social isolation and interpersonal conflicts • maintenance of friendships, intimate relationships, employment and appropriate recreational activities
Maintenance	• development of personal maintenance manual • mandated to attend maintenance sessions • support and encouragement	• attendance at maintenance sessions • acceptance of on-going risk • willing to disclose future problems which might put him at risk • allows significant others to discuss their concerns with therapist

as the offender thus becomes better able to appreciate the role deviant fantasy and cognitive distortions have played in motivating and overcoming their inhibitions to offend. In doing this, the offender's motivation to gain control over his deviant fantasies becomes enhanced and this increases the likelihood that he will comply with satiation and covert sensitisation training. Where deviant sexual fantasies are disclosed during assessment or in the course of analysing their offending behaviour, these need to be considered for early treatment through masturbatory satiation or covert sensitisation training. If deviant fantasies are initially denied, or when the therapist anticipates the offender will refuse to undertake satiation training, covert sensitisation can be introduced. Both these therapeutic exercises are valuable since they focus directly upon controlling deviant sexual arousal and the urge to sexually offend. Interventions focused on cognitive distortions, victim empathy and interpersonal skill training should, however, be delayed until the desire to offend is under control.

Analysing the cognitive behavioural chain of offending

Detailed examination of the thoughts, feelings and behaviour which lead up to a sexual assault, and the identification of those factors responsible for maintaining sexually abusive behaviour usually starts during assessment and continues as an early treatment focus. Whilst the analysis of this chain of events is a treatment objective, it also constitutes a further assessment procedure, identifying cognitive distortions, deviant fantasies and skill deficits which are subsequently the target of treatment intervention.

Treatment objectives

In examining the cognitive-behavioural chain (see Cycle in Chapter 1), there are a number of therapeutic objectives and desired outcomes.

The first objective is to remove the psychological defences: denial, minimisation, projection of blame, etc., which have been developed by the offender during the course of the abuse. Successful completion of this task may be indicated by an increased concordance of the offender's account of the sexual assaults with that of the victim.

The second objective is to identify in detail the process by which the offender moved to a situation of high risk and subsequently committed the abuse. For extra-familial offenders this process typically begins by 'befriending' a child or the child's parents. A relationship of trust is then developed, enabling the offender to be alone with the child and to test their response to surreptitious touching, before moving on to clearly abusive behaviour. Intra-familial offenders may begin the abusive process by, for example, sexualising conversations with the child, or by inappropriate touching at bath- or bed-time. Although treatment exposes such behaviour as planned and motivated by the desire for sexual contact with the child, the offender may initially attempt to rationalise, for example befriending a child, or having the child see him naked in the bathroom, as unconnected to the later abuse. Pithers *et al.* (1988) describe such events as being due to 'apparently irrelevant decisions' – AIDs, seemingly unremarkable decisions in the eyes of the offender, which are in fact expressions of his plans to abuse.

The treatment objectives include exposing such AIDs as significantly linked to the abuse and for the offender to accept his motivation and responsibility for making such decisions. When this treatment task is complete, the offender should be able to describe the cognitive behavioural chain of events leading to the abuse, accept responsibility for it and begin to recognise why certain behaviours must be avoided in the future if he is to remain offence-free.

The third objective is to identify those factors – e.g. use of pornography, seeing children he finds attractive – which have stimulated deviant sexual fantasies and desires, and those factors – e.g. social isolation, low mood, reduced self-esteem – which have disinhibited the sexually abusive behaviour. When this is achieved, the client becomes able to recognise these events as increasing his risk of offending and accepts the need to develop appropriate avoidance and coping strategies.

The final objective is to combine the above elements so as to predict future high-risk situations and their likely antecedents. When this objective is achieved the offender accepts that he is an ongoing risk, and can identify his high-risk situations. This, in conjunction with the development of skills to avoid or cope with risk, constitutes the essential elements of an individualised relapse-prevention package.

Exposing the motivations to offend

Treatment begins by providing the offender with a rationale for examining his offending behaviour and its relevance for future risk reduction. Victim statements need to be obtained before behaviour analysis takes place since these will contain details of the circumstances of the offences, the sexual assaults and provide a benchmark against which the honesty of the offender's account can be judged.

The offender is asked to describe in detail the events leading up to the first contact assault in the offending episode. Typically, offenders initially describe the assault and the events immediately preceding it and in doing so avoid admitting that before this they may have sexually fantasised about the child, given them special treats or attention, sexualised conversations and surreptitiously touched the child before the identified assault took place. Consequently the therapist needs to investigate events which took place over an extended period prior to the first assault, if all the relevant antecedent thoughts, feelings and behaviours are to be identified. Where pre-assault interactions between offender and victim are examined, the offender is asked to interpret the child's behaviour and his beliefs about the child's thoughts and feelings towards him. Such questions typically reveal cognitive distortions which may be challenged immediately or noted for later therapeutic work.

Progressively more detailed questions are asked until a coherent picture emerges regarding the offender's thoughts and feelings at each stage in the chain leading to the offence. Where offenders have difficulty, or resist exploring internal processes, for example, feeling sexually aroused, the therapist may offer a hypothesis to fill the gap and challenge the offender to provide alternative and more coherent explanations of his thoughts and feelings at the time. Homework can be set between sessions in which clients are asked to describe specific elements of their offending chain. This can also be used as a way of determining to what extent the therapeutic work has been understood.

When the abuse has taken place over an extended period, or where there is more than one victim, it will be necessary to examine several different cognitive behavioural chains before the full range of offence antecedents have been identified. This is important, since whereas one assault may be associated with low mood arising out of emotional isolation, another assault by the same offender may be triggered by the presence of a vulnerable child or by use of pornography, with low mood having an inconsequential role.

Developing avoidance and coping skills

Through detailed analysis of the offence antecedents it becomes possible to identify the way in which the offender gained access to children, the triggers and content of his sexual fantasies, the mood states which undermined his ability to control deviant urges and his distorted thinking, and how he planned to create the opportunity to abuse.

Treatment is designed to interrupt the chain of events leading up to an assault at the earliest possible stage, when the offender's problem-solving and coping skills are still intact and his urges to offend relatively weak. This is ideally at the stage where 'apparently irrelevant decisions' are made which result in increased contact with children. Not only must strategies be developed to recognise and avoid predictable risk situations, but offenders should also be trained to cope with, or escape from, unforeseen or unpredictable events which might undermine their self-control. This can be done by presenting the offender with a range of possible risk scenarios, brainstorming the range of possible coping responses and considering the pros and cons of each alternative solution. Since offenders frequently lack the behavioural skills necessary to put coping strategies into action, these should be rehearsed through role play to ensure he can translate intellectual understanding into behaviour. The ability to demonstrate problem solving and behavioural coping skills can be set as a criteria for treatment success. Following this training, agreed coping and avoidance strategies can be written on postcards and carried by the offender, placed on his car dashboard or pinned to the inside of his front door to serve as reminders on how to deal with risk. Where it is agreed that specific situations or behaviours should be avoided, these need to be shared with the offender's partner or others who will monitor his behaviour following treatment.

Depression and anxiety due to social isolation or interpersonal conflict are commonly reported by child sex offenders as mood states which increase the likelihood that they will seek association with children or as factors directly responsible for disinhibiting their urge to offend. For many offenders social isolation, low mood and poor self-esteem appear chronic problems and may require specific interventions in order to reduce the risk of reoffending. For some individuals, social skill training, improvement in dating and intimacy skills, combined with support, guidance and encouragement to develop less isolating lifestyles may be sufficient to enhance self-esteem and reduce vulnerability to depression. With other offenders this may need to be supplemented with interventions (e.g. Beck *et al.*, 1979), specifically designed to remove the underlying patterns of dysfunctional thinking which are responsible for causing low mood and low self-esteem.

Covert sensitisation

Covert sensitisation is a therapeutic training procedure which can be used by offenders to help interrupt the thoughts (deviant fantasies, day-dreams and cognitive distortions), and feelings (urges and longings) which cause risk-taking and offending behaviour. Training takes place in therapy sessions and the client practises the techniques as a homework assignment.

Treatment begins by identifying a chain of events which, on the basis of examining previous offending, might lead to a further offence. The positive consequences of avoiding relapse are then reiterated and a 'reward scene' is constructed which is personally relevant to the offender. This might be recalling a pleasurable experience from the past, or imagining a future reward for non-offending, e.g. being free of anxiety, having access to his children. This reward scene is used by the client when he imagines breaking the chain of behaviours which lead to a sexual offence. An aversive image is then constructed. This is preferably based upon previous painful consequences of offending – for example, standing in the court, hearing the charges read out, or the memory of being searched and deprived of possessions on arrival at prison.

The therapist demonstrates the treatment procedure by imagining and verbalising the behavioural chain leading up to an offence. The aversive image is introduced at a point where the offender enters into a risk situation but before the urge to offend is so high as to make an offence inevitable. The therapist then describes the offender escaping the risk situation and rewards this action by switching into the reward scenario.

Speaking in the first person, the client then undertakes the same procedure whilst being audio-taped. The therapist assists by prompting the client to attend to the details of the imagined behaviour and to the aversive image which is held long enough for the client to exhibit signs of anxiety or distress, before the escape route to the reward scene is taken. This procedure is then practised four or five times a week as a homework assignment, for a period of five weeks for each relapse scenario with audio tapes being returned each week for review. Several different relapse scenarios need to be targeted with most clients before training is complete. The homework can be extended into real-life situations by instructing the offender to bring the aversive image to mind when certain daily events occur which in the past have triggered risk-related thoughts or feelings. Such events may include seeing children he finds attractive, visiting friends with children or contemplating journeys past schools or playing fields.

As an alternative or supplement to covert sensitisation, offenders may be instructed to sniff smelling salts or valeric acid (a harmless, but highly malodorous substance), which can be carried by the offender in his pocket and used whenever risk-related thoughts or feelings occur.

Modification of deviant sexual arousal

Since such deviant arousal is considered to be one of the prime motivating factors in sexually abusive behaviour, its modification is a core component of many treatment programmes. The presence and focus of deviant arousal is determined either directly through self-report or by use of the penile plethysmograph, or through questionnaires, the analysis of sexual fantasy, and during the course of analysing the cognitive-behavioural chain of offending behaviour (see Chapter 3).

Treatment approaches

Aversion therapy and procedures designed to change masturbatory fantasies are the two main behavioural approaches to the modification of deviant sexual arousal. Since aversion therapy is a laboratory-based procedure which has fallen somewhat out of fashion, it will not be discussed further, though readers may refer to Quinsey and Earls (1990) for a review of its application. Of the four masturbatory reconditioning procedures available, none have undergone extensive clinical evaluation, though masturbatory satiation and directed masturbation appear the most promising procedures (Laws and Marshall, 1991).

Masturbatory satiation

Masturbatory satiation training is based on the assumption that deviant sexual arousal has developed as a result of the repeated pairing of deviant sexual fantasy and masturbation. The aim of treatment is to extinguish deviant arousal by breaking the link between masturbation and deviant fantasy. This is achieved through a combination of treatment sessions and homework assignments. Treatment begins with educating the client about the relationship between deviant arousal, fantasy and offending. The nature of appropriate sexual fantasies is then discussed; that they contain themes of mutuality and consent and deviant fantasies are identified for satiation training.

Homework

At least three times a week the client is instructed to masturbate to orgasm whilst focusing on non-deviant fantasies. Having ejaculated, and therefore reduced sexual arousal, he continues to masturbate and verbalise a deviant fantasy for a specified period. The complete exercise is audio-taped and the tapes are returned to the therapist for checking.

In selecting deviant fantasies or memories for satiation it is best to select a current fantasy, or one which was linked to the client's last offence. A succession of fantasies are targeted in sequence, and each one continued until it has lost its potential to arouse. Whilst generally the first fantasies targeted for treatment take the longest time to be neutralised, practitioners should be aware that offenders do not necessarily initially disclose their most arousing ones, keeping them 'in reserve' for when they need an extra stimulus. The amount of treatment time required varies between offenders, but often takes 20–30 hours of audio-taped work.

As treatment progresses, the significance of any deviant fantasy re-emerging is discussed, particularly as a sign of possible risk of relapse. The client is prepared for this possibility by making plans to cope (re-contacting therapist, initiating further satiation training), and is encouraged not to 'catastrophise', should deviant fantasies recur. This preparation helps ensure that such a lapse does not result in an abstinence violation effect (Marlatt and Gordon, 1985) whereby the client negates all the constructive progress he has made, becomes despondent and self-deprecating and abandons the coping and avoidance strategies he has learned to inhibit offending.

Dealing with cognitive distortions – reattribution training

Examples of cognitive distortion are gathered from a number of sources during assessment and treatment: cognitive distortion questionnaires, clinical interviews, analysis of the offending chain, victim empathy training and by examining the fantasies which are the focus of masturbatory satiation training (see Chapter 3). For offenders who report ongoing sexual thoughts about children, homework assignments can be set in which offenders are asked to bring back examples of events which trigger risk-related thoughts.

Therapeutic approaches

During treatment the therapist educates the client on the relationship between cognitive distortions and offending behaviour and challenges the way the offender misattributes children's behaviour and their intentions and feelings towards him. In doing this, the offender is pressed to acknowledge and understand the connection between his efforts to establish relationships with children, his underlying sexual interest in them and how this results in his interpreting children's behaviour in accordance with how he would like them to be: sexually interested in him, enjoying and not being harmed by sexual involvement with him, etc.

The therapeutic style is one of non-aggressive questioning and confrontation in which each component of an offender's statement is systematically examined for evidence of distortion, omission and misattribution. As statements and beliefs are selected for examination, the client is asked to provide evidence to support his belief or interpretation of events. Typically this approach reveals how a single offender statement may conceal several underlying misattributions of a child's behaviour or distortions of belief. For example, the statement 'the child did not tell because they enjoyed what they did with me' contains the assumption that the child enjoyed what happened, willingly participated in it and had the choice to disclose. When the theme of the child's sexual pleasure is explored, this may reveal how the offender misattributed elements of the child's behaviour. For example, he might suggest the child looked at him in a 'special way' which signalled sexual interest in the offender. This statement when explored may reveal further offender beliefs regarding children's high level of sexual knowledge and sophistication and how the offender believes society is misguided in condemning 'loving' sexual 'relationships' between adults and children.

It is not productive to challenge offending behaviour solely on the basis of its illegality – most offenders are already aware of this – nor on the basis of its being morally reprehensible, since offenders may reply that much individual and corporate behaviour breaks moral rules. The therapist should therefore be conversant with the short- and long-term negative effects of sexual abuse, be able to explain why children cannot consent (Abel, Becker and Cunningham-Rathner 1984b), be able to expose the offender's underlying motive to abuse and show the role distortions play in disinhibiting and maintaining sexually abusive behaviour.

As the offender develops his skills in recognising and challenging distorted thinking, he should be encouraged to remain aware of those children and circumstances which trigger such beliefs, to challenge the beliefs when they occur and to report back on his successes and difficulties in doing this.

Reattribution training can also be assisted by asking those offenders who have been sexually abused themselves to recall these experiences, to reflect upon how they behaved at the time, how this may have been misinterpreted, how their protests had been ignored, or stifled, whether they had consented, had enjoyed what happened, what had inhibited their disclosing and what had been the consequences of this abuse. Parallels can then be drawn between their own behaviour as a victim and those displayed by the victim of their own offence.

Role-reversal exercises may also be used to give offenders practice in verbally challenging distorted thinking. Here the therapist voices a distorted statement or account of a sexual assault and the offender is required to challenge those elements of the statements which he believes are distorted.

Emotional congruence

For some fixated offenders, cognitive distortion is associated with strong feelings of emotional attachment to and emotional identification with children. Such emotional attachments may be persistent even when deviant sexual arousal is modified and after skills in relating to adults have been improved. Consequently, such offenders must learn to accept these feelings as contributing to their ongoing risk of reoffending and must rehearse coping and avoidance skills to deal with these feelings. For some individuals, therapy may also be needed to help them cope with the feelings of loss and deprivation which are the consequence of relinquishing relationships with children who are for them so emotionally important.

Assessing change

Successful removal of cognitive distortions is evident when the offender is able to complete cognitive distortion questionnaires without error, demonstrate in role reversal exercises their ability to challenge cognitive distortions and can explain the role distortions played in their own offending behaviour. They also need to be able to identify their moods and the characteristics of children which trigger distorted thinking. Finally, they should be able to review their own masturbatory satiation tapes and explain which distortions are embedded in their deviant sexual fantasies.

Enhancing victim empathy

There is a considerable overlap between enhancing victim empathy and treating cognitive distortions, since it is only by the removal of distortions that the offender can fully allow himself to face the impact of his abusive behaviour. In treatment, offenders are assumed to have impaired empathy or to have developed techniques to suspend it, at least in respect of the victims they have abused. The two components of victim empathy training focus upon developing the client's intellectual appreciation of the impact of sexual abuse and applying this to their own victim, and, secondly developing their capacity for emotional sensitivity and responsiveness to victim distress.

Therapeutic approaches

During treatment the therapist directly educates and structures learning experiences which improve the offender's intellectual understanding of the damaging consequences of sexual abuse. Within treatment sessions, the client can be asked to watch video-tapes of survivors and victim therapists talking and to discuss how these relate to the experiences suffered by his own victim. Homework may include the offender reading books and articles on abuse, writing an account of their offence from the victim's perspective or answering questions which victims commonly ask their abuser (e.g. see Salter, 1988).

Victim apology letters may also be written and presented to the therapist or other group members for discussion and critical analysis. It is not intended that these letters be sent to the victim or their family, except following agreement with child protection workers who have vetted the letter and fully explored and considered the possible impact on those receiving it.

A victim apology letter needs to address a number of core issues before it can be considered complete. Such issues include the offender accepting responsibility for the abuse and distress and harm caused, an explicit statement that the victim was not to blame and was right to disclose, and an apology without expectation of forgiveness. Most clients have to rewrite their original attempt a number of times following therapist feedback and, in group treatment, from other clients. Not infrequently the initial victim letter not only omits to address important themes but also contains distortions which will need to be dealt with before a more adequate letter can be written. The following extract from a client's initial letter provides an illustration of this:

> The most important things I want to say to you are *sorry* and *no* hard feelings! . . . Now here's the most important part of this letter. Even though YOU asked me, you must blame ME for doing it – never ever blame yourself for asking. Grown ups are meant to know best and do what is right and I failed, didn't I? Certainly we're meant to know better than cheeky, pretty 9 years old with huge curiosities!
>
> You see not only did I like you very much, but I've always liked some young girls *too* much and that's why it happened. I was also very curious to know why *you* were so interested. You didn't say anything then but I know now you'd been playing special games.
>
> . . . Another thing that hurt me was your statement that you hadn't told for three years because you were afraid of me. We both know that wasn't true don't we? But how else could you explain about keeping quiet for all that time? . . .
>
> love Michael
>
> P.S. Have a good life. I'll never forget you.

Here, amongst other things, the offender denies his victim's harm and likely anger towards him ('no hard feelings') and continues to believe she was responsible ('even though you asked me'). He suggests the victim was sexually provocative towards him ('cheeky, pretty'), interested in sexual contact with him ('huge curiosity') and enjoyed sex with him. Furthermore, he denies any responsibility for ensuring the child's silence, suggesting instead that she had a choice as to whether or not to disclose. Finally, the overall tone of the letter is one conveying a continued preoccupation with the child.

Group therapy, discussed more fully in Chapter 5, provides the best setting in which to develop the offender's ability to emotionally appreciate the distress suffered by victims. Exercises in which offenders play the role of their victim and describe to other group members what is being done to them and how they feel about it provides a powerful means for 'getting in touch' with victims' feelings. In individual or group therapy, offenders can be asked to recount their own experiences of being sexually abused, not with the prime objective of working these feelings through (this may require separate therapy), but to examine their feelings and thoughts at the time and to compare these feelings with how their own victim is likely to have felt.

Assessing change

Successful enhancement of victim empathy is judged to have occurred when offenders are able to complete victim empathy exercises, demonstrate knowledge of the effects of sexual abuse on victims and write an appropriate victim empathy letter. Where treatment takes place and family reintegration becomes a prospect, the offender's willingness to meet with their victim, accept responsibility for the abuse and the victim's feelings about the abuse may also be set as a treatment goal (see Chapter 8). This face-to-face meeting may be preceded by the offender making a statement of apology on video for the victim to view. Only if the victim, the child's non-abusing parent and child protection workers feel it is satisfactory and free from victim blame and cognitive distortions should the meeting take place.

Social competence

Men who sexually abuse children often present with social difficulties, including social anxiety and avoidance, under-assertiveness, problems making conversation, and difficulties in sustaining intimate relationships and resolving interpersonal conflicts. Problems in social functioning are identified through a combination of clinical interview, questionnaires, direct behavioural observation and the reports of others (See Chapter 3). Whilst these problems are not unique to these offenders, they do help explain why many are lonely, have histories of intimacy failure and gravitate towards the company of children and young people who are less critical and more accepting than mature adults. There are several books and manuals detailing how to apply social skill training (e.g., Hollin and Trower, 1986) in addition to those which focus upon more specific areas of interpersonal functioning, for example, assertion (e.g. Liberman *et al.*, 1975) and anger management (e.g. Goldstein and Keller, 1987).

Therapeutic approaches

Social skills training (SST) focuses at both the micro level (e.g. eye contact, body posture, voice volume, interpersonal distancing), and the macro level (e.g. initiating, maintaining and ending conversations), of interpersonal behaviour. Stress reduction procedures are also utilised for clients whose social behaviour is impaired by or associated with anxiety.

Assertion training includes elements of SST and teaches both positive assertion (e.g. making requests, expressing appreciation or affection), which has a positive impact on the social partner, as well as negative assertion (e.g. making complaints, disagreeing), which has a potentially negative impact.

Anger management includes elements of SST and assertion training which are combined with specific training in preparing for provocation, dealing with confrontation and regulating the accompanying anger (Novaco, 1979). Where conflict exists in marital relationships and has been a factor contributing to sexual abuse, or where the offender's anger and aggression has prevented the non-abusing parent from protecting her children, marital therapy is included as a component of treatment. While the focus of these procedures varies, there is considerable overlap between them, and they share a basic training procedure consisting of problem identification and discussion, therapist instruction and modelling, client role play and feedback. Homework assignments are set between sessions to enable practice and skill generalisation to occur.

Whilst most of these procedures can be taught in individual treatment, a group format is advantageous since it generates a variety of perspectives and problem solutions. It also allows mixed gender co-therapy, to ensure training is as realistic as possible. Since some offenders are homosexual and avoidant of consenting gay relationships, heterosexual therapists need to be sensitive to clients' needs and should consider enlisting the help of gay counselling services and support groups.

Assessing change

Whilst change in social skills, assertion and self-expression is not uncommonly seen during treatment, such changes may be particular to the treatment setting and not necessarily be reflected in the client's daily behaviour. Consequently, in addition to self-report of success and therapist observation of improvement, it is highly desirable to obtain reports from other professionals involved with the client (e.g. hostel managers, child protection workers), employers, friends and partners to see whether they have seen similar positive changes. In reality, however, for those offenders who begin treatment as socially isolated individuals, the benefits of improved social competence: making friends, gaining employment, making and sustaining intimate adult relationships, may happen (if it does) over timescales longer than the period of therapy. This fact strengthens the argument for long-term maintenance, support and monitoring of offenders' progress.

Maintenance of treatment gains

Throughout treatment we need to impress upon offenders the importance of maintaining the gains they have achieved during treatment. Without maintenance programmes the impact of expensive treatment effort is likely to be lost. Consequently, not only should expectations of long-term contact be instilled in offenders, but where possible this should be specified in therapeutic, probation and parole contracts. Moreover, child protection agencies and the courts need to be encouraged to grant offenders access to their families, approve family reintegration, and the lifting of care and supervision orders, on condition that offenders agree to participate in long-term maintenance programmes. Practitioners, their managers and the child protection system need also to recognise, support and resource long-term arrangements to help offenders maintain their therapeutic progress.

Despite the recognition that sex offending is a life-time problem, there is little research or experience to guide practitioners and their agencies in deciding what is sufficient input to maintain treatment progress. This is unfortunate, given the cost implication of developing maintenance programmes.

Maintenance programmes which have been reported include the 'surveillance group' approach of Abel (1987), in which four or five people in regular contact with the offender monitor him after having met with the therapist to construct check-lists of at-risk behaviour and situations. Marshall *et al.* (in press) describes their clinic preparing lists of risk factors and coping responses with the offender prior to discharge, which the offender is instructed to carry at all times, to read periodically.

Each client is supervised on release by someone knowledgeable about relapse prevention who will intervene directly or refer the client to a community clinic, a half-way house, or at the worst, return him to the prison therapy programme. Other maintenance approaches include having clients return for periodic 'booster sessions' (Maletzky, 1990).

In the author's programme, maintenance sessions are planned to take place at approximately eight-weekly intervals in the first year after active treatment has finished. Thereafter sessions take place at three-monthly intervals. Sessions are focused upon those specific factors identified during treatment which might make the client vulnerable to relapse, e.g. how he has dealt with encounters with vulnerable children, managed interpersonal conflicts or a recurrence of cognitive distortions or deviant fantasies. Since relapse is commonly preceded by depression or anxiety, specific questions are asked about the recurrence of life events, personal setbacks and disappointments which might undermine his capacity to cope. Sessions not only review, but directly boost coping skills by, for example, role-playing problematic situations, and helping to challenge thinking patterns which contribute to low mood or which reduce self-esteem. Support, encouragement and guidance are given and a return to treatment or a change of living arrangements is not ruled out for clients at risk of relapse. For those offenders who have returned to their families, their partner is introduced to the basic principles of relapse prevention and is involved with drawing up signs of risk and risk-avoidance check-lists. Both she and the client are encouraged to make contact with the therapist between maintenance sessions if pre-agreed rules of behaviour are breached or they fear a relapse.

CONCLUSION

Given the complex needs of offenders, multi-disciplinary and multi-agency collaboration is essential if offenders are to be offered effective treatment and management. No single professional or agency has the skills or resources to meet all offenders' needs. Working with others helps ensure practitioners have the professional and personal support they need and enables the development of group work, family therapy and individual approaches, all of which are needed for comprehensive treatment.

The particular advantage of multi-agency work is in helping ensure the appropriate balance is struck between enabling offenders to change and rebuild their lives whilst ensuring that therapeutic enthusiasm does not jeopardise the protection of children. Moreover, working within a co-ordinated system helps ensure that resources are made available for long-term follow-up and maintenance.

In the final analysis, the degree to which offenders are treatable and whether they remain offence-free is dependent upon the interaction of many variables, including offender characteristics, practitioner skills, breadth of treatment, and availability of maintenance programmes. Given this, it is not surprising that treatment programmes vary in their outcome and that some abusers go on to reoffend. Marshall, Ward *et al.* (1991) have argued that even a modest reduction or delay in reoffending can represent a significant saving in human suffering and cost to society. Practitioners and managers need to accept the reality that some offenders will reoffend, and be prepared to deal with the ensuing criticism while striving to understand how they can improve their effectiveness in the future.

5   Groupwork with men who sexually abuse children

Paul Clark and Marcus Erooga

> The therapy of groups is likely to turn on the acquisition of knowledge
> and experience of the factors which make for good group spirit.
>
> (Bion, 1943)

INTRODUCTION

With the increasingly accepted orthodoxy of groupwork as the preferred
method of working (Barker and Morgan, 1993), it is important that
practitioners do not bring sex offenders together to work without having
explicitly considered the theory about effective groupwork as it relates to
this client group. In order to make best use of the opportunities they will
have created, and to minimise the potential risks, practitioners need to have
a clear understanding of groupwork theory in addition to their knowledge
about sex offender functioning.

Unfortunately there is currently no discrete theory of sex offender
groupwork. This chapter will, therefore, review key elements of groupwork theory and relate it to knowledge and experience of work with sex
offenders, illustrated with examples from the authors' own group
programme (Erooga, Clark and Bentley, 1990) in order that groupwork
with sex offenders can be planned and delivered with greater impact.

What do we mean by 'groupwork'

Before starting groupwork with sex offenders it is important to be clear
about the style of group required and its purpose. As the aim of working
with sex offenders is to develop increased responsibility for controlling
their sexually abusive behaviour, and given that their initial motivation
may be poor and levels of denial and distorted thinking may be high, the
choice of appropriate group models needs to take these factors into
account.

Brown (1979) identifies six models of groupwork practice, clarifying some of the major differences in aims and theoretical and practical emphases between the main types:

1 **Guided group interaction** Where the aim is to change delinquent and anti-social behaviour.
2 **Problem solving, task-centred and social skills groups** With an emphasis on achieving specific behavioural change in response to specific behavioural problems.
3 **Psychotherapeutic, person-focused groups** Concerned with individuals' emotional states and feelings. The main aim is to develop an individual's mental health, self-esteem and to strengthen interpersonal relationships.
4 **Self-help, mutual support groups** Essentially self-governing, with the focus on providing mutual support and help.
5 **Human relations training groups** Concerned with 'here and now' sensitivity training for those whose work involves them in group leadership and membership.
6 **Social goals groups** Concerned with groups in their social environment, differentiating between practical targets (e.g. housing improvements) and individual and social consciousness-raising and enhanced self-esteem.

PARTICULAR ISSUES IN GROUPWORK WITH SEX OFFENDERS

In determining the most appropriate model for this client group, it is important to consider the differences in working with sex offenders, as distinct from other client groups, adapted from those identified by Salter (1988).

Statutory vs. voluntary involvement

There are distinct advantages in statutory rather than 'voluntary' involvement in group treatment, albeit that 'voluntary' participants may not have a totally free choice, e.g. pressure from family or social services. Motivational levels often vary as circumstances change and offenders experience different pressures on them. Legally mandated attendance can serve to hold an offender to task and ensure continued group attendance. This does not preclude so-called 'voluntary' group members, but it should be recognised that there will most likely need to be significant negative consequences for non-attendance, as well as staff and peer expectation of an appropriate explanation for absences.

Explicit value stance

Workers need to have, or develop, a style of working that incorporates an explicit value stance. Although many practitioners are trained to adopt a non-judgemental approach to their clients, group leaders should not shy away from naming behaviours and attitudes as unacceptable, whilst ensuring that their approach does not become punitive and thereby counter-productive.

Confrontation

Confrontation needs to be based upon the provision of feedback:

> to help the client be aware of the nature of their thoughts and behaviours and reach a breakthrough – a genuine 'ah-ha' experience that illuminates the client's understanding of a concept and helps him to own the thought or behaviour in question. When confrontation is based in anger and shame and expressed through yelling, name-calling and put-downs, it may be a powerful experience that influences the client's thinking, but the change may be one that increases defensiveness and self-protection rather than understanding, by triggering the client's sense of victimisation, helplessness and poor self-image.
>
> (Ryan and Lane, 1991)

There is therefore a need for workers to find a style of working that holds these principles in balance – a style that balances respect for the individual without collusion, and one that holds group members to task through confrontation, whilst offering support at the same time.

Trust

Basing a relationship with an offender on trust is also likely to be problematic in that, even whilst the offender is endeavouring to be honest and straightforward, his distortions, self-deceptions and varying levels of motivation will make him an unreliable source of accurate information about his current situation, level of deviant sexual preoccupation, propensity to reoffend or past illegal sexual behaviour.

Confidentiality

Treatment needs to based on an explicit understanding that the extent of confidentiality is limited. Whilst a degree of confidentiality is important in order to provide a level of security to allow offenders to discuss their offending behaviour, this should be balanced against the needs of past or potential victims and the effect on current work. Maintaining the secrets of the abuse will not only be highly collusive and replicate the dynamics of the abuse itself, but can work against the process of offenders taking responsibility for their sexually abusive behaviour. From the outset it will need to be explicit that following group members' disclosure of further abusive behaviour or offences against other children, the information will need to be shared with the multi-agency network. This helps ensure that children can be protected and their therapeutic needs met, and also allows the offender to take further responsibility for his abusive behaviour. Considering the legal and ethical dilemmas arising from working with sex offenders, Goring and Ward (1990) conclude that 'consideration should be given to a Code of Practice establishing guidelines for the disclosure of information to those outside the groups themselves'.

Determining goals

At the outset workers need to identify goals and objectives for men in treatment. As offenders' motivation and understanding develop, they can become increasingly able to identify their own work goals and participate in planning, under the guidance of the staff group.

WHY IS GROUPWORK RELEVANT FOR THIS CLIENT GROUP?

Before considering a particular model for groupwork with sex offenders, it is necessary to consider why groups are a particularly relevant medium for therapeutic change. Reviews of current treatment provision show that the majority of programmes include some element of groupwork, with a significant number of programmes being based entirely on groups. Indeed, Barker's survey of Probation Service provision found that 'Treatment is offered by Probation Services largely through groupwork . . . [which] is felt to be the most effective way of working with sex offenders' (Barker and Morgan, 1993).

Behroozi (1992) suggests that groupwork is the preferred method of intervention for involuntary clients, as the group experience can reduce levels of denial, facilitate an acceptance of the fact that their problems exist, increase their need for change, and help clients to develop more appropriate ways of dealing with their problems. He also states that, due to issues of trust and authority being problematic with involuntary clients, confrontation which addresses the sources of their denials is far more effective when undertaken by their peers – all factors very relevant in work with sex offenders.

Secrecy

Commenting on the potential of groupwork for all those affected by sexual abuse, Glaser and Frosh (1988) assert 'Groups offer particularly suitable settings . . . in large part due to the central defining characteristic of a group, the collective aspect, which offers an alternative experience to the isolation, secretiveness and shame that is central to child sexual abuse.' Groups therefore inherently facilitate overcoming the secrecy which is likely to have pervaded the sexual offending, and offer the opportunity to begin to accept the new social identity of someone who has sexually offended against a child which their abusive behaviour now demands.

Motivation

Although many sex offenders express a desire to enter into treatment and begin a process of change, this is often at a time of crisis, for example following arrest and prosecution, or whilst being denied contact with their children. Consequently, their motivation to enter into treatment is often for externalised reasons and, given a free choice, many would not chose to do so. In this sense they should be considered to be what Behroozi refers to as 'involuntary clients' even when they are expressing apparently high levels of motivation.

Offenders' motivational levels are also variable (see Phases of change, below), as reflected in the fluctuating strength and changing nature of their denial. Behroozi suggests that the reluctance of involuntary clients such as sex offenders is a defence motivated by their frustration stemming from three sources – being coerced into change; having different perceptions from others about the nature of their problems and of their need to change; their pessimism about the achievability of the change targets. Thus even the most motivated of group members can experience extreme pressure to withdraw from the group when the work becomes difficult.

Adam was cautioned by the police for his offences of indecent assault against his stepdaughter. This decision was partly based on his genuinely contrite presentation and expressed desire for help. He expressed strong motivation to attend the group, both because of his distress at having offended and in order to work towards increasing contact with his own 7-year-old daughter, with whom he had weekly contact, supervised by her mother. Having made good progress in the group, he asked permission to go on holiday with the child and her mother. He was asked to consider between sessions the confusion for a 7-year-old of this temporary change in the pattern of contact. His response was to consult the child about her view, which attracted considerable challenge from the group. In the face of this he absented himself from sessions. His stepdaughter subsequently disclosed further details of the extent of his abuse of her, for which he was then prosecuted and re-referred to the programme. Following further assessment, he rejoined, subject to a probation order with a condition of attendance – a more appropriate legal response than the initial police caution.

Yalom (1975) has identified a number of 'curative' factors in what he describes as 'group psychotherapy': instillation of hope, universality, imparting of information, altruism, recapitulation of the primary family group, development of socialising techniques, imitative behaviour, interpersonal learning, catharsis, existential factors and group cohesiveness.

These are summarised below with reference to their applicability to groupwork with sexual offenders.

Group cohesion

The primary and most important curative factor, for Yalom, is group cohesiveness, the 'attractiveness of a group for its members; . . . what keeps them [engaged] in the group'. This is seen as a precondition for effective treatment. Whilst compulsion may be the external motivation for joining a group, successful members will remain because of the attractiveness of the group, and because of what they derive from the group. This attractiveness enhances the group's reinforcing value, thereby encouraging members' change of attitudes and behaviours. A safe, secure, but not confidential, environment provides a context in which members can share sensitive information about previous abuse or current fantasies or behaviour (e.g. compulsive masturbation), or about factors which may have hindered previous change. It also provides a setting to deal with powerful emotions and socially taboo issues, again a particular feature of work with sexual offenders. The group allows for the increased use of experiential methods (e.g. role play, art and dramatherapy). Such techniques can be used very productively to explore feelings that are more easily suppressed and controlled in individual work. Group support also enables members to ask questions of themselves and others which it would be hard to ask in one-to-one settings. Although individuals get less exclusive attention in groups, they do afford the opportunity to learn from the experience of others.

Universality

During initial contact many sex offenders describe a sense of uniqueness which can inhibit attempts to seek, or participate in, treatment. Group process can address this by what Yalom calls 'universality', the experience that they are not alone but that others have faced, and continue to face, similar problems. Having overcome their initial anxiety, many men in groupwork report this as one of the most positive initial benefits of attending a group: 'I realised I wasn't the only one who had ever done this, and that others felt bad too.' The group also allows members to see problems, attitudes, feelings and behaviours similar to their own from a safe distance, enabling a more objective focus on their own issues.

Altruism and instillation of hope

Groups of people with similar problems may share very similar needs and can, therefore, provide a valuable source of mutual support and mutual approaches to problem solving. Often it is this sense of acceptance which leads to the capacity to make life changes (Belfer and Levendusky, 1985).

'Altruism' refers to the help that members provide to each other by way of positive group interactions. This is doubly beneficial as it will not only require members to 'step back from their own pain to offer support to fellow members' (Belfer and Levendusky, ibid.), but also enables members to feel valued for the contribution they are making. Brown (1979) describes every group member as 'a potential helper'. Each group member can, by relating their own experiences to the solution of other members' problems, act as a source of help which can often serve to cast them in a role that they have hitherto either not perceived or not experienced, and can serve to enhance the helpers' self-image and self-worth.

Brown also identifies a prerequisite for change as being therapeutic optimism by the group members – their belief that change is possible. Instillation of hope occurs as new members experience the support of their fellow group members and observe others improving and changing. Expectation of success is a major factor in positive outcomes and, as the timescale involved is likely to be longer than initially anticipated by most participants, the sensitive management of members' expectations will be an important task for leaders (see Phases of change, below).

Feedback and modelling

A key benefit is the process by which the group fosters changes of attitude and behaviour through feedback and modelling. Of particular relevance to sex offenders is Sullivan's theory (1953) that, based on life experiences, individuals may develop inaccurate cognitions and unhelpful responses with regard to interpersonal relationships. These distortions will emerge in the group, which then gives the opportunity for them to be identified and commented upon. In addition, members can observe more functional social models, practise new social behaviours and obtain coaching and feedback from the group, activities which are described by Yalom as 'imitative behaviour' and 'development of socialising techniques'.

Brown similarly identifies that as most people experience membership of different groups in their social lives, whether it be family, work or leisure groups, a formed group can be an effective medium to work on interpersonal and social interaction problems in order to subsequently generalise their learning and gains in other social situations.

Recapitulation of the family group

Yalom suggests that the origin of relationship problems may lie in experiences from early family life which can be addressed by the group process. He says that problematic early interactions can affect current interactions in the group, through transference, and the group can serve to recapitulate (or replicate) the primary family group, thereby working on exposing the source of the social interaction problem.

> Bill struggled socially to be assertive and reported that in past relationships he had not been able to express his feelings openly and that this had led to him bottling up his emotions, with frequent explosions of destructive and abusive rage. In the group he presented as emotionally flat, and often avoided conflict, ascribed to his difficulty in expressing his feelings in other situations. The group leaders progressively directed the group to be aware of their feelings and the relationship of feelings to their behaviour, as well as to hold the group to task in order to face up to conflicts between members. Bill was able to learn how to deal with his feelings, initially inside the group and subsequently outside in his social network. He reported back to the group with some satisfaction that he had avoided a situation in a shopping centre where he once might have responded with anger and violence. He said that he had been confronted publicly by a one-time neighbour who knew about his sexual abuse of his daughter. He said that once he might have retaliated when pushed and jostled but reported moving away without exacerbating the situation and without using violence. He was able to talk in the group of the feelings of anger at being confronted in this way, and how he had been able to recognise the problems he would have caused by retaliating and how he had 'watched himself dealing with this angry man' where once he would have struck back.

Generalisation

A central process of groupwork is generalisation – the sense each offender is able to make for himself from considering other members' experiences in the group. Without this process, groupwork can be little more than one-to-one work in a group setting. The latter might be evidenced by an over-concentration of time on one individual, and by group leaders acting as a 'switchboard' for all communication in the group, providing little opportunity for other members' comments or connections being expressed. Without the verbal expression by group members of this connection, workers can only hope that such connections are being made.

> Chris expressed concern in the group that the behaviour of his 13-year-old son, David, was becoming more rebellious and difficult for his wife to handle on her own at home. He was allowed supervised contact with David but his son chose not to attend, because he found the restricted contact difficult. Chris spent time outlining his feelings of power-lessness at being unable to influence this situation. As he spoke, his sense of depression was felt in the group, and in turn each of the other group members identified their own similar feelings as they outlined their own restricted contacts with their families. Although none of the group members were able to offer a concrete solution to Chris's problem, they were able to validate his feelings and help him gain new insights into his situation in a way that also focused the rest of the group on issues and feelings related to the consequences of their offending behaviour.

In this way one man brought an issue relevant for all the group which each worked on in their own way. Those men who did not contribute were prompted to do so and thus became involved in the generalisation process.

Having recognised the advantages of groupwork with sex offenders, the question arises as to which model of groupwork is the most appropriate to use with these clients.

A MODEL FOR SEX OFFENDER GROUPWORK

Given the complex nature of work with sex offenders, groupwork practice with sex offenders will inevitably be eclectic, usually containing elements of the first two models outlined by Brown (1979) (guided group interaction and problem solving, and task-centred groups). A strong focus should be given to developing group members' abilities to deal with their own feelings in appropriate and non-abusive ways. Experiential methods are a particularly valuable means of achieving this. In managing the group, there will need to be flexibility between time spent on group tasks and attention to group process issues. Self-help, i.e. members helping each other within the leader-led group, should play a part in the group process but should not become a central theme or groupwork modality. There will be some degree of an educational component and, in mature groups, members should be expected to bring their own specific issues to the group to work on, under the guidance of the group leaders. Additionally, given the complex impact of sexual abuse on family networks, treatment will need to be undertaken with any partner and other family members, in conjunction with a long-term groupwork component.

Belfer and Levendusky (1985) describe this approach as long-term process-oriented behavioural group psychotherapy, with the goals accomplished 'through a combination of members' learning to identify problem areas, applying relevant behavioural intervention, and increasing the probability of compliance to these interventions by fostering a group process that then holds each member accountable.'

Many of the approaches to intervention and treatment are similar to those used in individual treatment as described in Chapter 4, and are summarised below.

Treatment components

Sexual assault cycle

Group members need to work on developing and presenting a verbal account of their abuse, using the assault cycle structure to focus their thinking. Other members give feedback on aspects of minimisation, cognitive distortion and denial. At each stage of the cycle, members should identify what they were doing, thinking and feeling.

Cognitive distortions

Initially members may need to have an explanation of the term 'distorted thinking' and to develop their understanding of the purposes it serves. Similarly they may need to have the functions of minimisation and denial explained to them. Group members need to identify examples of their own cognitive distortions, and need also to be able to recognise and challenge those of other group members. Learning from other sections of the programme, e.g. victim awareness, is a vital part of this work.

Sexual arousal

Focusing on offence patterns can serve to develop an understanding of group members' sexual arousal patterns. This work is not designed to alter sexual fantasies, but rather to gather more information about them. Work on fantasy modification (referred to in Chapter 3) may require individual work quite separate from the groupwork programme. Caution should be exercised in coming to premature conclusions about the extent of illegal sexual arousal patterns. Being aware of the possible extent of offenders' denial and minimisation should warn against such early assessments.

During the assault cycle work, members need to acknowledge and identify masturbation fantasies, patterns of sexual arousal and masturbatory fantasies used during the period of offending. They also need to identify current masturbation fantasies, as well as current patterns of sexual arousal. Some of this work can be developed in the group session, providing the basis for individual homework assignments between sessions.

Sexual history

Generally, this will be completed as an individual homework assignment in the form of a sexual autobiography, which may take a considerable time to complete. One of the aims of this is to allow the offender to explore aspects of his sexual development and consider how they have impacted on his offending behaviour, attitudes, beliefs and fantasies.

Victimisation experiences may be raised in group sessions and these will need to be linked with their own abusive behaviour, rather than focused on directly in the group. Where an individual's victim experiences have caused them to block the associated feelings, they may become stuck when trying to consider and connect with the feelings of their victim. Overcoming fear of arousing their own suppressed emotions and working on their own victimisation may be crucial to improving victim empathy. It may, however, be necessary to provide, or arrange, separate victim-focused work for group members. This may raise very real ethical issues about whether or not to insist that a victim undertakes therapeutic treatment.

Sexual issues

Group members' awareness of the purpose and function of sexual behaviour and sexuality will need to be explored, as will identification of areas of 'sexual ignorance'. Linked to this can be an exploration of what, and how, non-sexual needs have been met by sexual means. For example, Wolf (1984) describes masturbation as a stress management technique for sex offenders. Therefore the non-sexual function of the abuse needs to be explored when considering group members' offending patterns and antecedents.

Feelings

Group members will need to understand the link between feelings, thoughts and behaviour and to identify ways they have blocked feelings, or how having one feeling can be a defence against others – what Berne (1975) describes as 'rackets'. A 'feelings diary' can serve to focus attention and may need to be completed over a lengthy period of time.

Victim awareness and victim empathy

Whereas victim awareness is an intellectual process, victim empathy describes the emotional connection with the victim experience. It will be important not to confuse the two, as whilst awareness may soon be learned, there may be considerable emotional investment on the offender's part to resist making the more difficult connection. These separate aspects may be most effectively addressed in different ways. Awareness may require a didactic approach, whereas empathy may be best achieved through experiential techniques.

Victim awareness can explore issues of the rights of children as individuals; children's perspectives and experiences of the world; power and consent issues with victims, why children cannot give consent (Abel, Becker and Cunningham-Rathner, 1984b); understanding damage to victims of abuse; understanding effects of specific aspects of members' behaviour on their victims.

Victim empathy can be enhanced through the use of experiential exercises that allow the offender to experience the victim's experience as near as is possible, without it becoming an abusive experience in itself. This may require careful preparation of the group before each exercise.

Exercises may include gestalt 'chair-work', mime, artwork (painting, collage) and any other technique which may access the victim's experience on other than a verbal, intellectual basis.

Attitudes to women

Group members may express attitudes to women that are as unacceptable as their attitudes to children, and which will need to be challenged directly. There are often implications as to how the group members relate to female members of the staff team and it will be important for the whole team to pay attention to these processes to avoid collusion with such attitudes.

Relapse prevention

When an offender understands his own cycle, he should then be able to share this knowledge with his partner, or relevant others, by developing his own partner alert checklist (North West Treatment Associates, 1988). He needs to understand all aspects of his cycle and the implications for his feelings, thoughts and behaviour, as well as the relevant implications on his victim and his partner at the time. Group members should develop a relapse prevention plan with identified triggers, danger situations and strategies to cope with these prior to leaving the group.

Social skills

It may be appropriate to include a specific component on social skills acquisition. However, as most sex offenders have misused their inter-personal social skills in the commission of their offences, it is important to ensure that provision of social skills training is not based on a misapprehension about the reason for sexual offending. Without increasing victim awareness and empathy, enhancement of social skills for this client group can present the risk of developing a more socially skilled offender.

No component in the groupwork programme will be entirely self-contained or concluded as a theme before moving on to other components. The feelings component, however, may need to precede victim awareness work, as self-awareness of feelings is the basis for victim empathy.

PLANNING FOR EFFECTIVE GROUPWORK

When planning to run a group for sex offenders it is important for group leaders to understand the relationship between the structural aspects of the group, selection, contracts, etc., and how these impact on the process of change for the group members. For a group to be effective, issues such as selection criteria, group size, as well as an understanding of leadership tasks, which will all affect the establishment of a therapeutic environment, must be considered.

Korda and Pancrazio (1989) identify several leadership characteristics and practices that can serve to limit the potential negative outcome in groups in general. They suggest that particular consideration should be given to screening and preparation of group members, establishing a safe environment, managing conflict, dealing with transference and counter-transference, and limiting negative effects should they occur.

Screening and preparation

On selection and screening, they point out that 'pre-group training or orientation is helpful in both decreasing the incidence of dropping out and in increasing appropriate group participation'. It has been our experience that having a rolling programme with a periodic 'feeder group' to the main treatment group facilitates new members joining more experienced members and allows them to become more rapidly integrated into the group and the norms previously established. It is important therefore for group leaders to develop a shared set of criteria for the selection of group members, which should be centred on an understanding of motivational levels and their ability to function in a group.

Group agreements

The establishment of a safe environment will depend on leaders initially paying attention to defining ground rules and member–member confidentiality. Member–leader confidentiality issues should have been defined in an individual agreement prior to involvement. It will also be important to be clear that challenging feedback is different from hostility, and a shared commitment to respect for all members and leaders. Korda and Pancrazio (op. cit.) suggest that 'inappropriate group pressure is less likely to occur with a leader who models an attitude of acceptance, caring and understanding', which it is possible to achieve without collusion with members' distorted thinking.

The issues of control likely to be presented by this client group, and the sensitivity of issues to be dealt with, suggest that establishing member–member agreements, starting and finishing on time and having rituals to open and conclude each session (for example, a round of feelings) will help increase the 'safety' of sessions by providing a structure for meetings. This safety will help establish a 'therapeutic environment, open and honest communication, member–member support and sharing as well as establishing the group as a place where members change and grow' and that these are established 'through interventions by the group leaders in the very early sessions' (Belfer and Levendusky, 1985).

Managing conflict

Conflict is an inevitable stage of a group's development and will need to be dealt with in order to move towards a cohesive and effective group which is able to work together. The way in which both positive and negative feedback is given and received can affect levels of group conflict. Korda and Pancrazio note that it is important for leaders to model appropriate ways of both giving and responding to feedback.

Subgroups and pairings can also have a negative influence on the group, and Yalom suggests that group leaders need to actively discourage such relationships, indeed to pay explicit attention to it and make it a group expectation or norm that no socialising occurs after the group or between sessions. A further reason for this is the recognition that offenders may well support each other's minimisations and distortions when not being challenged by the rest of the group or the group leaders. These reasons should be fully explained to group members, and this may require particular attention with sex offenders in prisons and hostels (see Chapter 6).

Transference and counter-transference

Yalom suggests leader strategies to cope with transference (in which the client responds not to the worker as they are, but to a stereotype connected to a previous relationship (Mattinson and Sinclair, 1979)). This requires group leaders to exercise fair treatment for all members, to encourage verbal expression of feelings and needs in order to 'dispel belief in leader omniscience', to encourage group validation of individual perceptions of group leaders, and to demonstrate leader congruence as well as appropriate leader self-disclosure.

Counter-transference (workers' unconscious response to the transference, e.g. becoming aggressively angry to a particular group member) can be dealt with by leaders paying attention explicitly to their own needs in pre-and debriefing with co-workers or in supervision, and using recordings of sessions to review their own ways of responding to particular group members. Korda and Pancrazio suggest that leaders' negative attitudes to group members, and the consequent adoption of such attitudes by group members, may be more effectively dealt with by workers involved in co-leadership.

Limiting negative effects

Negative outcome in groups can be limited by paying attention to skills and preparation of leaders, professional compatibility of co-leaders, paying specific attention to feelings when members join and leave the group, and minimisation of leader absences (Korda and Pancrazio, op. cit.). In addition, if leaders share a value base, an understanding of theoretical issues relating to sex offenders, the process of change and group dynamics, this will contribute to a strong staff team better able to establish a cohesive groupwork environment.

IMPLICATIONS FOR PRACTICE

Yalom identifies the main tasks of the group leader as being the creation and maintenance of the group and the establishing of group norms. In order to accomplish these aims, particular issues will need to be attended to.

Group norms

At the outset, group leaders will need to overtly establish, and monitor, group norms in order to produce an environment which is conducive to positive change. Group leaders will initially be the prime agents of unification for the group and members will initially relate to the group through the leaders, especially during the first stages of flight and fight (see below). Over time this will change, and as the group develops cohesiveness, members' relationships to, and within, the group will become less dependent on the group leaders, resulting in much more member-to-member interaction. Attention also needs to be paid to establishing anti-offending norms and language, not least the expectation of disclosure rather than denial. Yalom identifies an important task of group leaders as being to 'deter forces which threaten group cohesiveness', such as lateness, non-attendance, member–member attacks, and disruptive extra-group socialising as some of those negative forces (Belfer and Levendusky, op. cit.). Early in the life of a group it is important to establish the use of 'I' statements (e.g. 'I get angry when people disagree with me', rather than the more generalised 'You get angry when people disagree'. Encouraging the use of 'I' means beginning to take responsibility for feelings and views expressed. It will also be important to encourage specificity rather than 'safer' generalisations.

Giving and receiving feedback are skills that may need to be learned by group members, but provide a way of structuring important dialogue to best effect and provide the expectation that behaviour will be commented on. Related to this will be establishing a group commitment to appropriate peer confrontation, particularly challenging distortions and minimisations.

Content vs. process

A key issue for practitioners is how they balance the focus between content and process issues during group treatment. Content deals with the group subject matter, tasks and explicit focus of the group. Process relates to the underlying group dynamics, interactions and developmental phases. It deals with the tone, atmosphere, conflict/cooperation and often submerged feelings that exist in the group that are not always openly dealt with. Group workers who maintain the focus on the content without paying attention to the process will deny themselves and the group members the opportunity to explore interpersonal and group dynamics and feelings that will be essential to assist the process of change and to assist the group through its developmental phases: 'The behaviour group therapist constantly grapples with the alternative needs to emphasise proven behavioural interventions with the need to emphasise the curative factors of the group. In the dynamic tension that is created, effective treatment occurs' (Belfer and Levendusky, op. cit.).

During an introductory group programme, or the early sessions of a long-term group, there may be a greater emphasis on education/information giving, combined with modelling and fostering appropriate group behaviour. In the longer term, however, it is important for the work to be undertaken at a feelings level, both to reduce rationalisation and to provide emotional support in dealing with painful and personal issues. It is not uncommon for offenders to resist this by maintaining their group experience at an intellectual level, thereby avoiding the more difficult and painful components of change.

Action methods

Sustained change will only be based on changes in underlying beliefs, attitudes and behaviours. Whilst intellectual appreciation is therefore important, this needs to be coupled with a deeper emotional change. Such changes may necessarily be accompanied by a degree of emotional discomfort. In addition to discussion, 'action-methods' can serve to allow group members to experience their, possibly previously suppressed, emotions and encourage, as well as giving the opportunity to rehearse, the new behaviour.

Mixed gender working

Given the complex demands on those leading groups of this nature, mixed gender co-leadership offers the best opportunity to maximise the potential of the group, and reduce the possibilities of collusion or deflection and minimise potential negative effects on staff (see Chapter 9).

Preparation and consultancy

Group leaders may also benefit from developing structures to assist them in the complex task of running the group. These include adequate preparation and attention to leadership issues by allocating time for briefing and debriefing. Consideration should be given to the use of live consultation, a third worker observing the group session who may offer suggestions by telephone link and make observations during any break and after the session. By remaining uninvolved, the live consultant is often able to offer a unique perspective to the group leaders and to make suggestions about strategies for intervention.

Group leaders may also wish to agree that if they feel stuck or are experiencing significant difficulty, they will take a break during the session to consider the problem (Masson and Erooga, 1989). Having agreed this as a possibility before any problem arises, and advising the group that this may be done, makes its use more likely and less dramatic.

As well as live consultancy, many staff groups find benefit in the use of periodic meetings with an outside consultant, with whom they can review group functioning, staff group issues and programme content planning, as well as team building and maintenance and any personal issues that arise.

Recording

It is important to have a structure for recording the focus and process of the group work sessions. Different agencies will have different expectations of the nature of records, but they will all demand that some level of recording is completed. Recording fulfils several functions. It details sufficient information to inform others of the work that has been undertaken in each session and it allows for accountability by the agency or agencies concerned. In the process of recording, group leaders can debrief sessions and identify the integrity of the planned treatment, i.e. determine whether the work planned was the work that was delivered in the group.

STAGES OF GROUP DEVELOPMENT

It is our experience that groupwork with sex offenders can be effective in developing motivated individuals, able to focus upon effecting changes in their behaviour, thoughts and feelings. However, workers need to understand the processes of group development if they are to maximise the opportunities for real change that exist in group treatment.

It is not sufficient for groupworkers to leave this development to chance. Agazarian and Peters (1981) note that 'unless there is a specific input to stimulate group growth, the passage of time does not guarantee progression' and conclude that time alone may act as a force for creating a fixated group which is incapable of real change. They state that there are specific approaches and inputs that workers need to adopt to ensure a dynamic and developmentally healthy group process. Central to this is an understanding of the phases of development which occur in long-term groups, also highly relevant to long-term group work with sex offenders.

Writing from a psychotherapeutic perspective, they identify six phases of group development: flight, fight, power and authority, overpersonal enchantment, counterpersonal disenchantment, and interdependence. These stand alongside, and perhaps elaborate upon, Tuckman's (1965) rather more catchily named 'forming, norming, storming, and performing'.

The first phase – flight – is focused upon issues of joining and being included in the group, and is where the dynamic force is described as 'dependence and the wish for conformity', with group members overdependent on leaders, leading towards conformity to group rules and norms. Flight is described as an essential beginning phase of group development, in that it exemplifies the avoidance of difficult work in the group. It is at this defensive stage that members may pair with another group member to form a collusive relationship in order to confound the group workers and other potentially challenging group members.

The second phase – fight (counterdependence) – centres on seeking to regain control by using disruptive tactics to avoid situations where the group member feels challenged and confronted with the real task of change.

> At their first group session Doug and Eric realised that they knew each other, having lived in the same neighbourhood and having also served parts of their prison sentences in the same prison, where they had told each other they had been convicted of offences of dishonesty. Having overcome their initial surprise, they began to develop a strong alliance based on angry and intimidatory challenges to other group members in order to deflect direct challenges to themselves. They would attempt to sit beside each other and would make excuses for each other's behaviour and attitudes in the group. Each knew the strength of the other, and this attempt at collusion also served, in their own minds, to protect themselves from direct challenge from each other. This pairing had a strong impact on the group process and was one that had to be confronted directly. The pairing process, its function and effects, had to be named by the workers, and other group members empowered to also intervene. Once openly identified, it became increasingly difficult for Doug and Eric to sustain this behaviour.

Scapegoating, a common group process, is identified as the 'overt manifestation of the fight phase, with competitive subgroups scapegoating each other, an issue or a particular member' (Agazarian and Peters, 1981), as in the following example:

> Eric had been sexually abused himself yet had not begun to work on issues of his own victimisation. During work on victim empathy issues, Frank acknowledged his similar experience, Eric responded with anger and hostility, accusing Frank of making excuses for his offending and trying to enlist the sympathy of the group. This was in contrast to the perceptions of the group leaders and seemed to be designed to make the group an unsafe place in which to explore issues of group members' victim experiences, thus avoiding having to address what were for Eric very painful, and still suppressed, feelings.

Agazarian and Peters' third phase revolves around issues of power and authority, of developing relationships and alliances both for support and for 'contention and disagreement'. The central power struggle at this stage focuses on the members' relationship with the group leaders, but it is also the time when group members build their levels of solidarity and when the 'uninitiated therapist may mistake this sudden group unity for groupwork, and congratulate himself [*sic*] and the group for having resolved the dependency that they had been manifesting such a short time before in flight and fight'. In fact at this stage the group is not 'working' but is reconstituting itself to perpetuate the struggle for authority and control. As control and misuse of authority itself are central to the dynamics of sexual offending, this is therefore a key issue both within the process of group development and for individual members.

> Just as the authority issue is an experiential crisis for the group, so it is for the therapist. The entire group must be ready to work through the relevant dynamics. Sometimes the therapist is ready and the group is not. Sometimes the group is ready and the therapist is not.
>
> (Ibid.)

At this stage there is a danger that group leaders are so controlling that they do not allow the development of the group process, in particular the expression of authority issues.

The fourth phase is described as 'overpersonal enchantment' – seeing the group as Utopia. Characteristically, group members work on issues independently of the group leaders, and in this phase the assistance, support and help of the group leaders is not actively sought. It is because group members may feel very comfortable at this stage that there is the risk of the group becoming stuck. 'Should the group reach a level of equilibrium in this state, there is group fixation', although given the high levels of energy required by members to maintain this position, it cannot be maintained. 'As the work of the group centres more closely around maintaining the euphoria rather than expressing it, "closeness" becomes "too close"'. At this stage, group leaders must take steps to move the group on or risk collusion. This can be particularly challenging as it may be one of the first times leaders do not feel criticised by members for lack of progress.

The response to these steps is the fifth phase – counterpersonal disenchantment – which is characterised by distrust, fragmentation and frustration with the group. Conflict returns, cohesion is disrupted and the group is precipitated into a phase of disenchantment.

In the final phase – interdependence – the group has developed a healthy state of trust between group members and is ready to work on therapeutic goals corporately. The group has become strong enough to 'recognise characteristics of earlier phases when they recur. It has a memory of successful methods that have been used in working through phases and the experience of previous mastery of vicissitudes in development'.

In relation to long-term behavioural groupwork, Belfer and Levendusky summarise that 'The goal is accomplished through a combination of members learning to identify problem areas, applying relevant behavioural (and cognitive) interventions, and increasing the probability of compliance to these interventions by fostering a group process that holds each member accountable.'

INDIVIDUAL CHANGE IN A GROUP ENVIRONMENT

Central to any work intended to bring about change in behaviour is a conceptual understanding or model of how change occurs. Prochaska and Di Clemente (1982) have suggested a very useful general model of change, outlined in Chapter 2. During groupwork with sexual offenders the authors have identified a series of phases which appear to be part of the process of individual change with this client group, a process that relates well to the Prochatska and Di Clemente model. This is helpful both in understanding their responses in the group and in preventing premature optimism by workers about progress in treatment. It should be borne in mind that whether the member's initial motivation is an explicit desire to control sexual offending behaviour, or simply to be allowed to return to live with a family, there is a considerable incentive to be seen to be successful in treatment, and this is reflected in the phases.

The model is a flexible one and clients may not exactly follow the sequence described here. As identified in Chapter 1, during the compulsive assault cycle, some offenders' feelings of guilt about their abusive behaviour are likely to be intensified and prolonged, following discovery and intervention into the abuse. These offenders are therefore more likely to initially present as described in Phase two, rather than Phase one.

PHASES OF CHANGE

Phase one – *denial and resistance*

Even those men assessed as appropriate for groupwork may continue to deny or minimise aspects of their abusive behaviour. Their denial may focus on quantitative elements of the abuse – possibly the frequency or duration, or qualitative elements – the nature and extent of the abuse, or both. This denial serves as a self-defence mechanism to protect their self-image and preserve a view of the world designed to present their behaviour in the most acceptable light and to avoid, or reduce, guilt and responsibility. This distorted thinking prevents insight and defends against the feared, probably painful, consequences of facing the reality of their behaviour, being honest, the resultant effect on their self-image and esteem and the demand to relinquish their behaviour and change.

Phase two – *guilt and false motivation*

This phase is usually characterised by an initial presentation of remorse, guilt, embarrassment, self-pity and possibly preoccupation with the further consequences of discovery – break-up of the family and public shame, exposure to the criminal justice system and possible custody and loss of employment. This often creates a high level of compliance in the group – what might be described as a desire to please in order to be seen as somehow 'cured'.

This is essentially false motivation. It also leads to unrealistic expectations about the nature of their problem and the extent of the changes needed; about the timescale of treatment ('I just want to be home for Christmas'); and about the chronic and entrenched nature of their offending behaviour ('All this has been so awful, it will never happen again'). These views, naive though they may appear, are often sincerely held, and may persist despite attempts to provide a more realistic perspective. This may be a lengthy phase and one in which workers have to guard against responding to the client's sincere avowal of desired change, rather than measuring his actual progress.

Phase three – *awareness and compliant resistance*

The onset of this phase is characterised by an intellectual awareness of the issues and the beginning of an understanding of the work which needs to be undertaken. In our experience it is often work on victim awareness issues which has a powerful impact on group members. It can move forward thinking from a self-focus and breach the barriers and distortions they have created to block out the effects of their offences on their victim. The consequence of this is a shifting of balance in their motivation from a priority to return home/reunification, to seeing the need for treatment in order to avoid relapse, though both elements of motivation will still be present. What is often observed is a parroting of 'correct' responses; in effect, more and better compliance, which is often combined with praise of the group leaders. Underlying this, initially, is the absence of comprehensive or detailed understanding of the issues, or genuine acceptance of personal responsibility, though the desire to be different will be the basis of future work. This can indicate that new perceptions are beginning to become internalised.

Phase four – *awareness and internalisation*

This is when distorted beliefs are owned and core constructs change, rather than responses being repeated, the offender having learnt that they are correct. Given the long-term nature of the work, early progress towards this phase can be ruled out, despite appearances to the contrary. This phase represents genuine and sustainable changes of attitude and beliefs and is difficult to evaluate in the short term. It will be evidenced by a greater willingness to tackle painful emotional issues associated with facing up to the full extent of their responsibilities and the damage done to the victim and other significant relationships. Evidence of real change in behaviours as well as attitudes will need to be sustained over a period of time, and is likely to be a cumulative process, marked by indications of progress and slipping back.

Phase five – *awareness and responsibility*

This is the point at which, having successfully negotiated Phase four, and therefore having effected real change in their core beliefs and behaviour, renewed contact with, or rehabilitation into, a family can begin to be considered. It should be expected that the offender will now be actively taking responsibility for being aware of his own cycle and triggers, and for alerting professionals if he feels he is at risk of relapse. There will also be an acknowledgement by the offender that the risk of relapse is lifelong. The focus of work will now be on relapse prevention work for the long-term and developing rules for living, concerning relationships with children and partners, jobs, leisure pursuits, etc. These activities, along with making relevant others aware of potential warning signs, will be central.

Throughout the treatment process men may get stuck or fail to progress beyond early phases. They may also demonstrate a different rate of progression through the phases in connection with different aspects of the work. Their feelings of anger may prevent them from even beginning treatment, or contribute to this 'stuckness'. On the other hand, it will be important not to equate apparent motivation, or sincerely expressed remorse or desire to change, with change itself. It is the misinterpretation of motivation which most commonly gives rise to over-optimistic 'assessments' of future risk, in which offences are described in terms such as 'isolated aberrations – not likely to happen again'.

The phases of change can be seen in the case of George, who pleaded guilty to indecently assaulting his 10-year-old stepson, and received a suspended prison sentence. Whilst living separately from them, he maintained a relationship with the child's mother, although the court had ordered that he should have no contact with his stepson. At court and subsequently, both mother and child had said that they wanted George to return home.

George presented as an articulate, sincere and very plausible man. At the time of prosecution and sentence he was dealt with in a way which served to minimise his perception of the seriousness of his abuse and the risks he presented. The pre-sentence report described George's behaviour as 'totally out of character'. In his application to join the group, George stated that he was doing so to convince the Social Services Department that he was no longer a risk and to effect a return to his family. However, during pre-group assessment interviews he demonstrated some ability to acknowledge that he had been sexually aroused during the assaults and that they had not 'just happened' as previously asserted.

He was advised that the group leaders did not share his perception of himself as being no further risk, and that if he joined the group he would be expected to work on the full range of issues in the group programme. His view was that 'he had nothing to hide', and he agreed to participate fully in the group. Despite his stated motivation for joining the group, there was evidence of movement and he expressed willingness to work on the relevant issues. Consequently George was offered a place, albeit with some doubts about how long he would stay.

At the initial contracting meeting the social workers involved with the family identified the work they were planning to undertake with George's partner and stepson – separately and jointly. Any future involvement of George in this family-based work would depend on his progress in the group and on future court decisions regarding contact.

His contract specified that there should be no contact with his stepson either directly – through visits or telephone calls – or indirectly – by third parties, letters, etc. Social Service's view was that the child was feeling responsible for the separation of the family. Contact with George, because of his distorted views of his offending, was not likely to help the child at this stage.

In his first group session George contradicted statements about sexual arousal made during assessment and reverted to presenting himself as no risk *(Phase one)*. He spoke of the court welfare report, the pre-sentence report, the probation officer and magistrates all wanting him to return home to his family and said that he had joined the group in order to effect a return home as soon as possible.

In subsequent sessions his preoccupation with the urgency of his task frequently led him to try to force the pace of his treatment, by focusing on promoting himself as no longer presenting any risk *(Phase two)*. Consequently he resisted fully understanding the past, present and future effects of his abusive behaviour on his stepson.

Although superficially socially accomplished, George's self-esteem was in fact low and he was emotionally flat. Apart from anger, he struggled to distinguish between his feelings and his thoughts, which he was keen to express, especially as they usually concerned his perceptions of the continuing damage being done to his family by the professional system. Because of his own emotional flatness he was unable to understand his stepson's feelings, so that victim awareness and empathy were seen as key pieces of work for him to undertake. Initially the other men in the group also saw George, who was the most articulate of the members and the most socially accomplished, as an exception, a nice man who had made an isolated mistake. However, over time, with intervention and challenge in the group by staff, they began to challenge George's position.

After four months, George began to identify his cycle of abuse *(Phase three)*. Now, rather than denying sexual arousal to his stepson, George was able to identify how he had begun thinking sexually about him prior to any abuse, and how he had arranged the opportunities to abuse him.

In his work in the group, George tended to regard his understanding of each issue as meaning he had 'solved that problem', still seeing the abuse as an isolated aberration *(back to Phase two)*. After 12 months' work George appeared to be fully engaged and from his own work, and the feedback he was able to offer others, he seemed to have begun to make some fundamental changes in his thinking *(Phase four)*.

It was at this time that he informed the group that he and his partner were expecting a child. When he learned that a child protection case conference was to be convened to determine the response to this development, George became very defensive and threatened to abscond with his partner before the baby was born, and abandon his stepson. Over the ensuing weeks he reconsidered his initial reactions, which prompted an intensive period of victim-focused work in the group. Though the staff group were disappointed at having over-estimated George's progress, he was subsequently able to develop his perceptions about the likely effects of abandonment on his stepson and seemed to make particular progress in developing his victim awareness *(Phase four)*.

In individual sessions he began to understand how his childhood experiences had contributed to his adult behaviour, particularly in his relationships with women. He now understood how he had been entirely self-centred, with a disregard for anyone else's feelings and needs. He undertook experiential exercises to link the feelings evoked with those of his victim – a springboard from self to victim. Other work included artwork and creating collages about attitudes to children, women, victims and about feelings. He then returned to his sexual assault cycle work to integrate new understandings and continued his work in the group.

In relation to the phases of change, George had moved from Phase one (denial and resistance), through Phase two (guilt and false motivation) and into Phase three (awareness and compliant resistance). By this point he had an intellectual grasp of the issues involved, but any changes at an emotional level were not sufficient when his own needs were most acute. Consequently, when tested in crisis, he demonstrated that his attitudes and behaviour were still to be fundamentally affected and in fact he was merely responding correctly verbally, without a real change in the level of his understanding.

Although George's story can be read as an example of the difficulty of working with sex offenders, it can also be seen to demonstrate the importance of testing the extent of change over a long period of time, under the pressures of real-life stresses. This applies to all sex offenders undergoing any form of treatment, either groupwork or individually based. Additionally, it emphasises the need for long-term groups to address the entrenched attitudes and patterns of behaviour that sex offenders present.

CONCLUSION

In this chapter it has been suggested that, in order to maximise the effectiveness of service delivery in groupwork with sex offenders, it is important that workers combine their knowledge about sexual offending with an awareness of the developmental phases of groups, as well as the phases of individual change. It is suggested that the model of groupwork outlined offers the maximum opportunity for effectiveness, and will ultimately be based on careful preparation of group structure, participants, and the staff team. Professional issues are considered further in Chapter 9, but an adequate basis for co-work will include a shared knowledge base about sex offenders, a shared value base, shared understanding of the theoretical knowledge and basis of change in long-term cognitive-behavioural groups, clarity about the programme and skills to undertake the methods and techniques. Daunting though this list may appear, the authors' experience of running, and consulting to, groupwork programmes with sexual offenders is that these goals are achievable and that ultimately groups can offer a unique opportunity for change to sexual offenders.

Finally, it is important to consider the most frequent criticism levelled at groupwork with sex offenders: how can we know whether it is effective? This is a developing area of work, and whilst the Home Office sponsored STEP research programme (Beckett *et al.*, 1994) provides useful and unique information about groupwork interventions in the UK, it is relatively small-scale and in the long term there is a need for ongoing research and evaluation to systematically attempt to determine what works. We owe it to victims and offenders to provide a service that is as effective as possible.

6   The management of sex offenders in institutions

David Briggs

It is all too easy to overlook the potential for therapeutic work with sexual offenders within institutions. It has long been asserted that our institutions simply enhance the deviancy of inmates; but we do not have to accept this premise, and it is timely to encourage those working within institutions, such as prisons and Special Hospitals, to strive towards the goal of offence-focused intervention and rehabilitation for those offenders who are motivated to control their behaviour upon release. This chapter describes secure systems, alongside a discussion of those influences which impinge upon the sexuality of those incarcerated and addresses some of the key issues in the assessment and treatment of incarcerated offenders. Following discussion of training issues for staff it concludes with suggestions for the 'next steps'.

THE SPECIAL HOSPITALS

The Special Hospitals, of which there are three in England (Rampton in north Nottinghamshire, Broadmoor in Berkshire, and Ashworth near Liverpool; Carstairs Hospital serves Scotland), include sex offenders amongst their population. They are designated to provide treatment, under conditions of special security, to those mentally disordered patients deemed to require such on account of their dangerous, criminal or violent propensities.

For an application for admission to the Special Hospitals to be successful, it must be proven that the patient is liable for detention and is also dangerous. Thus, the person in respect of whom the application is made must be detainable under the 1983 Mental Health Act as suffering one of those types of mental disorder defined in s.1 of the Act, namely severe mental impairment, mental impairment, psychopathic disorder, or mental illness. Furthermore, if the person suffers from mental impairment or psychopathic disorder, that person is only detainable if treatment is likely to prevent a deterioration in that person's condition or is likely to alleviate the condition.

The definition of 'dangerous' can be problematic, with the phrase 'grave and immediate danger' usually taken as the benchmark against which decisions are made. In considering what represents grave danger, particular behaviours or patterns of behaviour are significant. These include sexual assaults on members of the public, delusional beliefs focusing on specific people which could lead to the patient committing violent acts against them (e.g. a frenzied sexual murder), and sadistic behaviour.

Statistics detailing a breakdown of the Special Hospital patient population as a function of their offence type or problem behaviour are not widely published. Dacey and Butwell (1991) of the Special Hospital Research Unit have provided details of the Special Hospital sex offender population for the period January 1972 to December 1987. These figures represent those patients housed within the English Special Hospitals during that period, but exclude the Carstairs population.

Overall, sex offenders constitute approximately one-third of the total Special Hospital population. Murrey *et al.* (1992) has undertaken a preliminary investigation of the sex offender population at Rampton Hospital. The case-notes of 106 sex offender patients were analysed for this study, representing clients with a Mental Health Act classification of psychopathic disorder, mental illness and mental impairment. These patient groups were compared across a number of variables: age on first

Table 6.1 The Special Hospital population, 1972–87

Offence	Number of patients with the offence recorded as the index offence at time of hospitalisation	Number of patients with the offence recorded in their history but not as index offence
Buggery or indecent assault upon a male	132	76
Rape or attempted rape	201	87
Indecent assault on a female	268	308
Unlawful sexual intercourse	19	(Not reported)
Gross indecency with a child	21	(Not reported)
Indecent exposure	(not reported)	94

Source: Special Hospital Research Unit 1991. With acknowledgement to Dacey, Butwell and Taylor)

documented sex offence, intelligence at admission as measured by the intelligence quotient or IQ, sex offence type, frequency of offending, history of violence during sex offences, and number, age and gender of victims.

The results of the survey revealed that 88 per cent of sex offender patients suffering psychopathic disorder and 98 per cent of mentally ill sex offender patients offended against female victims. Some 56 per cent of the mentally impaired patients' victims were female. Of the victims of mentally ill and psychopathic patients, most were pubescent or adult females. The victims of the mentally handicapped patients were primarily males or females under the age of 16 years. IQs correlated positively with a history of violence during sexual assault, and mean IQs were higher for 'violent' than for 'non-violent' offenders in each offender category.

Caution must obviously be exercised in drawing conclusions from such surveys. The usefulness of this study lies in the prompt it provides for the development of theories about sexual offending. The mentally impaired sex offender population has been neglected by researchers, leaving a series of unanswered questions. Why is it that our mentally impaired patients are more likely to be convicted of abusing males or young children, and use less violence in their assaults? What are the characteristics of mental impairment (if any) that influence the *modus operandi* of sexual offending? Do our institutional practices and policies exacerbate the potential for some clients, more than others, to reoffend?

INSTITUTIONAL INFLUENCES ON SEXUALITY

It is disconcerting to the practitioner working within institutions to perceive that the sum total of institutional influences upon the inmate's or patient's sexuality is negative rather than positive. Cooke *et al.* (1990) have described the psychological effects of imprisonment. They highlight the concept of 'loss', namely loss of control and choice, loss of family, loss of stimulation and, importantly, for sexual offenders, loss of pro-social models.

Consider, for example, the case of the incarcerated rapist. Social learning theories of rape emphasise learning by observation. Rape is construed as a facet of aggressive behaviour toward women. The potential rapist is hypothesised to assimilate images of violence towards women, including explicit rape scenes, from observation of such in the media or in real life. Repeated exposure to such stimuli desensitises the observer to the unpleasantness of the material: pain, subjugation and distress lose their salience. The distinction between sex and violence becomes blurred when these images are shown in the same context. The observation of sexual violence, within pornographic films, for example, is often accompanied by the modelling of excuses and rationalisations for the behaviour by sexual aggressors.

Regrettably, characteristics of the institutional environment *also* offer unhelpful models of adult sexuality. Some prisons in particular have an inmate subculture of violence where aggression is not only a survival tool, but a mechanism for enhancing status, obtaining privilege and channelling frustration at the depersonalisation of prison life.

Aggression here includes sexual aggression. This may be manifest in behaviour ranging from forced masturbation, through forced fellatio to buggery and gang rape. It would be naive to assume that such activity is not visible. Indeed, as part of the power hierarchy, other inmates may be called upon to 'stand guard' to avoid discovery of the abuse. The point to be made is simple. Such activity provides just that negative model of the fusion of sex and violence that social learning theory would postulate as important in the genesis and maintenance of rape behaviour.

Needless to say, we are more comfortable as a professional community in examining the sexual assault of inmates and patients by their peers than contemplating the same being committed by staff. Inevitably, given the nature of institutions (with the relative isolation and depersonalisation of inmates, and the imbalance of power between inmates and staff), and the motives of a small number of people to work in such institutions (knowing that institutions can provide opportunities for the satisfaction of abusive emotional and sexual drives), abuses will occur. This must be faced and dealt with by the managers and staff of our institutions alike.

The modelling of sexual violence is but one of several crucial aspects of institutional life influencing the inmate or patient's sexuality. Issues of homosexuality, sexism and pornography also require discussion.

Sexual orientation

Homosexuality raises strong emotions in many workers within our institutions, emotions and attitudes ranging through fear, anger, distaste, benign acceptance, curiosity and titillation. Myths concerning homosexuality are easily identified and are as relevant to the sexuality of staff as to that of inmates and patients.

The successful management of sexual offenders cannot occur, however, without proper consideration of the offender's sexual orientation. Whether a person is sexually attracted to an adult of the same or opposite sex (or both) may or may not have a functional relationship to their sexual offending proclivities. Too often, the expression of homosexual feelings within institutions is taken to be indicative of poor sexual control *per se* and hence indicative of likely relapse upon release. Even within the past decade, treatment goals have been targeted at 'helping' the sexual offender develop consenting, sexually functional, heterosexual relationships with adult females, regardless of the client's sexual orientation. Our clients readily assume the language of the converted heterosexual: 'All I want to do when I get out of here is settle down, get married and have kids.' There is no ethos of acceptance of non-heterosexual orientation within many institutions, and consequently staff cannot respect the legitimate homosexual orientation of the inmate or patient. The problem is compounded by a culture which will neither encourage nor enable staff (of whatever discipline) who are homosexual or bisexual to share this with their professional colleagues. This has personal consequences, let alone in their work with clients.

The law relating to sexual behaviour is often used to justify institutional policy. Section 1 of the Sexual Offences Act 1967 provides that homosexual acts between two men over 21 years of age are not illegal, if they are in private. Hospitals and prisons are not deemed to afford privacy within the meaning of the Act. Whilst inmates are unlikely to be prosecuted if found having such relationships, the response is unlikely to be supportive or encouraging of their behaviour. Obviously direct care staff have a responsibility to ensure that those in their care are not victimised or abused by others. The management of consenting homosexual relationships poses difficulties for most staff, including those ultimately responsible for clients, and consistency of approach within institutions is rarely achieved. We can speculate that the denial by staff of their own and their clients' sexualities leads to denial of other issues important in the rehabilitation of offenders.

Sexism and sexual displays

An interesting difference between prisons and Special Hospitals is the display of pictures of naked women (or occasionally men) in many prison cells, not so prevalent in hospital side rooms and wards. Cowburn (1991) in his study of sexual offenders in British prisons noted differences between male and female workers' awareness of issues pertaining to sexism. Men presented with more 'confined' and ambivalent views as to what was sexist and how sexism impinged upon their work, in contrast to female workers who reported sexism within institutions and its negative impact on their personal and professional lives. Silence about the issue, or humour, were used to cement the sexist ethos, which both male and female staff felt powerless to change.

It seems clear that even those highly motivated to work constructively with sexual offenders can be ambivalent towards these issues. Workers express a range of concerns: male workers' fears that women might be able to do a better job than men; the feelings that if male and female staff are to be integrated, then other staff and clients will compete for female attention and hence disrupt the smooth running of the unit; some male workers' beliefs that female staff need to be protected. The pessimism of individual workers that such beliefs cannot be changed seems to be reflected in the inattention or inability of managers of some institutions to confront these issues.

Influences on fantasy

Critics of the prison system have long argued that imprisonment does little to rehabilitate the perpetrators of sexual crime, but does a lot to consolidate and reinforce their illegal interests. The main sexual outlet for most incarcerated sexual offenders is masturbation, with the use of external stimuli and internal imagery (sexual fantasy) to enhance arousal.

George and Marlatt (1989) describe the fantasising about sexual offending as representing a lapse situation for those offenders who are trying to control their behaviour. They argue that for those offenders who are incarcerated, the attachment to their offence pattern can be maintained via fantasising at very high levels, and by masturbation to those fantasies.

Within institutions there are many opportunities for the sexual offender motivated to feed his fantasies of illegal behaviour. In addition to photographs depicting infants and children in magazines and newspapers, children feature regularly in television programmes. Newspapers can provide lurid descriptions of sexual crimes involving children, though such reports do not compare with the rich detail provided by the written statements of those involved in the trials of sexual offenders. Such written descriptions of offences are often available to prisoners when pre-trial defendants, and may be kept by them following conviction.

Those incarcerated within institutions have opportunities to discuss their sexual interests in children with other like-minded individuals. We should not ignore the opportunity that group therapy affords sexual offenders to hear details of other's sexual behaviour, material which will be arousing to some and can be incorporated into fantasy unless the group therapists challenge this and afford opportunities for their clients to control their fantasising. In this regard, institutions are not sterile environments; indeed, some might argue such environments are anti-therapeutic and supportive of pro-offending attitudes and behaviours. For rehabilitation to be effective, the content and control of their sexual fantasy life will have to be addressed for all offenders.

THE ASSESSMENT OF CLIENTS IN INSTITUTIONS

The overriding consideration within secure hospitals is the assessment and controllability of risk. The issue is particularly relevant for those patients who are housed in Special Hospitals. Decisions about the transfer or discharge of those patients will be made on the understanding of a resolution or stabilising of the patient's mental state, and those patients no longer requiring care or treatment within the conditions of high security afforded by the Special Hospitals. In practice, these criteria are fused under the global concept of dangerousness. Hospitalisation is indeterminate for Special Hospital patients – the knowledge of this may be a motivator for those clients whose mental condition allows such insight. It has to be remembered that a significant number of patients in Special Hospitals who have a sexual offending history may be difficult to assess in respect of their dangerousness, owing to fluctuations in their mental condition, or deliberate intent (which may or may not stem from their mental condition) to fabricate information upon which decisions about dangerousness are made.

The most commonly used assessment tool is the clinical interview. Comment has been made in earlier chapters on the dilemma of self-disclosure for the client. Kaplan (1985) has emphasised the relationship between the confidentiality of the interviewing situation and degree of self-disclosure in paraphiliacs. Offenders in our prisons and Special Hospitals do not enjoy confidentiality within those institutions; we must respect the problems of the validity and reliability of information obtained from clinical interviews conducted in these settings.

Regardless therefore of mental condition, the patient has to resolve a dilemma: that of deciding the depth or quality of information to offer the care team about his offence history. Of most help to the assessor are full details of the frequency of previous offending, including offences not prosecuted, the developmental pattern to offending, and the content of each offending episode, including details of planning or sadism involved, and the nature of the client's fantasies. Such detail, however, may raise fresh concerns in the immediate assessor, or others involved in the decision-making process about discharge or transfer.

Psychophysiological assessment

The use of penile plethysmography is not widespread within prisons and Special Hospitals in the UK at this point in time. Abel and Rouleau (1990) highlight difficulties in the psychophysiological assessment of sexual arousal for incarcerated persons (the measurement of penile responses to types of sexual stimuli). Specifically, the prisoner or patient who is aware that information derived from such assessments is to be used to assist parole or transfer decisions, in their opinion, is likely to be motivated to suppress their deviant sexual arousal and to hide the extent and form of their sexual interests. We already have evidence that some Special Hospital patients can suppress sexual arousal to preferred images, or enhance arousal to non-preferred images when instructed to so do (Briggs, 1979). Thus, data from psychophysiological assessments should not be used in isolation when making decisions about discharge or transfer. Nor can such an assessment tool be used retrospectively to determine whether an inmate or patient has committed a particular act, as the penile plethysmograph has no validity as a lie detector. Erection responses are thus best used either within clinical practice with motivated patients to determine treatment needs and gauge treatment outcome, or in research.

The Home Office Prison Department initiative

In November 1990 the Home Secretary announced a major initiative for the assessment and treatment of adult male sex offenders in prisons. This was initially based on the development of co-ordinated treatment programmes to be run in 13 prisons, selected to specialise in this work. Staff working in those establishments were to be given special training; opportunities for support and professional development were to be encouraged. Senior management within establishments agreed to prioritise resources for these projects, and the initiative was to be monitored and evaluated centrally from the Home Office Prison Department.

Two main treatment programmes have now been established (Thornton, 1991). A core programme is designed to address offenders' distorted beliefs and excuses. Work is additionally targeted at the development of victim empathy, the offender learning to take responsibility for his offending behaviour, and the offender understanding the likely relapse process and thereby considering relapse prevention strategies. A second programme runs for men considered to be a higher risk, though this currently applies in only six institutions. In this 'extended programme', deviant sexual arousal is a focus, as are communication, anger and stress management skills.

Thornton (1991) has identified the principles upon which the assessment of inmates for these programmes will be based. These are the use of multiple sources of information to reduce bias in the assessment process, the use of a systematic and objective process of assessment, the careful training of those involved in assessing inmates to maximise consistency in observation and judgements, the use of clinical skills to obtain information, and the use of a statistical formula based on research and expert advice to integrate information. Sources of information will include a medical/ psychometric assessment, details of the inmate's behaviour on the wing, psychological tests including penile plethysmographic assessment of sexual arousal, clinical interviews and group sessions concerning offending cycles, the recorded history of convictions for sexual and violent offences, and information concerning life circumstances outside the prison (both current and as pertained at the time of the offence).

Priority for inclusion in the two programmes are those serving sentences of four years or longer; the scope of the challenge is underlined when it is considered that this is a population of some 2,000 inmates. The programme has emphasised an empirical approach throughout, and an evaluation of this project will represent one of the most important pieces of UK-generated research in this field for many years.

THE TREATMENT OF CLIENTS IN INSTITUTIONS

Prior to the development of the co-ordinated strategy for the treatment of sex offenders in custody, sex offender treatment in prisons was a marginal activity. Like contemporary community-based programmes, the prison programmes were dependent on the enthusiasm of individual staff members (often probation officers), they were vulnerable to shifts in resources, were not centrally co-ordinated and did not permit monitoring and evaluation at a local or national level. Treatment content and emphasis varied across institutions. Lack of training for staff, wide variations in staff attitudes towards this client group and organisational problems within institutions also contributed to the problem.

Within Special Hospitals similar considerations apply. Members of the hospitals' clinical teams may offer group-based or individual therapies to sexual offenders, and treatment will be co-ordinated by the patients' responsible medical officers. However, at the time of writing, there are no wards or units which specialise in the treatment of sexual offenders as a discrete group.

Given contemporary debate about the effectiveness of treatments for sexual offenders (Marshall, Ward *et al.*, 1991) and difficulties in applying predictors of recidivism to the individual case, treatment programmes on offer to clients within institutions will, of necessity, be eclectic and potentially over-inclusive in character. Furthermore, the programmes offered should best be considered as precursors to longer-term treatment and follow-up in the community or less secure establishments. It would be dangerous to assume that the majority of persistent sex offenders leaving our institutions could function independently without longer-term follow-up, aftercare and monitoring. Worryingly, we face the potential collapse of therapeutic gains made in institutions, due to lack of resources and expertise in aftercare.

'Menus' for therapeutic interventions in Special Hospitals can be considered, similar to those described by Thornton (1991) for the prison sex offender programme. Several important points should be made, however:

1 Prior to work being directed at aspects of the offence behaviour, it will be important to motivate clients to engage in therapy. Clients should be clear as to why they need to change their behaviour and how their lives will differ as a consequence of these changes; therapists should understand constraints upon change, should understand whether clients believe they can change, and should articulate clearly how change will be promoted and managed. This motivational work might be set within the following pathway:

Reception into the institution

|

Assessment

|

Motivational programme

|

Educational programme

|

Other therapeutic programmes

|

Relapse prevention preparation

|

Transfer from institution

Within this scheme it is suggested that offenders following assessment and motivational treatment should enter an educational phase. Here, they can be given information such as that detailing the laws relating to sexual behaviour, be offered education, and be given details about the management of their case and exit criteria for leaving the institution. The educational programme is then followed by treatment packages covering training in victim empathy, social and assertiveness skills, anger management training, and awareness of cycles and patterns of offending. Both group-based and individual therapies are likely to be involved at this stage, ideally with the involvement of both male and female therapists. Prior to transfer from the institution it is suggested that preparatory work on relapse prevention be undertaken, such as that described by Laws (1989). Given that the thrust of relapse prevention is on maintenance strategies for pro-social behaviour post-treatment, this work will inevitably be developed and refined at other treatment programmes which, hopefully, offenders will attend when released or transferred. Although this scheme places assessment as an independent early stage in the process, obviously assessment will be ongoing throughout the scheme. Some offenders will require re-entry to the motivational programme as new therapeutic challenges arise.

2 Experience of running treatment programmes at Rampton for mentally impaired patients and those patients suffering from psychopathic disorder suggests that the effectiveness of therapeutic packages is compromised unless opportunity is also given to the patients' to address non-sexual offending issues. The importance of befriending, support and encouragement to these client groups should be emphasised. There is a need to integrate the attitude, behaviour and skills change strategies mentioned above with other factors known to help clients change. The honesty and integrity of workers and their genuine respect for clients should be encouraged.

3 The management of denial often poses particular problems for workers dealing with offenders in the institutions. Denial is an inevitable feature of offender work. This should not surprise us. Workers are often helped in their management of denial if they are encouraged to consider clearly the nature of the phenomena. As discussed in previous chapters, denial is not a trait fixed in the offender, but rather is expressed within a relationship between an interviewer and client. It may take many forms, and may be motivated by a fear of negative consequences – for example, owning the unpalatable truth of the distress the perpetrator has caused victims, a fear of retaliation from family or friends, a fear of abuse from other inmates, or fear of being unable to change. Statements of denial or minimisation might be modelled on the behaviour of others. Some offenders might enjoy power over the interviewer through their persistent denial. The effective management of denial will be dependent upon a proper understanding of the motivation for such (see Chapter 3).

Examples of interventions

Often workers in institutions feel powerless to intervene with inmates, feeling that the odds against successful therapeutic work are stacked heavily against them. We should view these difficulties as challenges. Some of our most creative work has been generated within institutional settings. For example, the subject of motivation is very relevant to the incarcerated population. This can be tackled directly, using a series of structured questions as topics for debate and discovery with our patients:

- Why is it important that I change?
- Do I believe I have the ability to change?
- What does change really mean – what will I have to do that I don't do now; what will I have not to do that I do now?
- Who can help me change, and in what way?
- What have I tried to do in the past to change? – why wasn't it successful?

A decision matrix can be used to help our patients consider the short and long-term consequences of change. An example is given in Figure 6.1.

In the example it can be seen that the response is a very egocentric one; little thought is given to the issue of future victims or harm to others. It is important to work this through. In this example we would be keen to explore why the patient has difficulty acknowledging value in not re-offending, for himself and for potential victims.

Simple tools such as the decision matrix can yield very rich rewards as spring-boards for future discussion and the monitoring of attitudes. The most effective style will be honest (i.e. not minimising the difficulties of change, the potential for lapses, or the uncertainties of institutional decision making), challenging (non-punitive), facilitating the client's thinking (rather than thinking for them in a traditional institutional manner) and caring (to provide a model of non-abuse interaction).

Offenders with learning difficulties

One of the most exciting challenges that faces us is the adaptation of

| | Short-term consequences | | Long-term consequences | |
	Positive	Negative	Positive	Negative
To change	It will please my key worker	I get scared because I might fail	I'll get out of this place	I'm going to have to stop doing things I really like doing
Not to change	I will be able to avoid some real hard work	The staff will give me hassle and pressure me	I can keep on doing risky things, but I'll have to be careful not to get caught	People won't let me live my own life – they'll always be watching me

Figure 6.1 The decision to change – an example of a decision matrix

materials and techniques for patients with learning difficulties. The majority of patients with learning difficulties are not literate. Traditional flip-chart work with words to summarise key points within group sessions are of little help. Visual symbols are more potent. For example, if attempting a behavioural analysis of an offence, cartoons of the patient and key players can be used as literal representations of the sequence of actions. If the patient cannot draw too well, other group members can be encouraged to help. Sessions about victim effects subsequent to offending again can use pictures to help, e.g. drawings of a crying face to depict depression, of a frightened face to depict fear, and so forth. Psychodrama techniques offer an alternative medium for work. Experience of work with the learning difficulty client group suggests:

- the need for relatively brief (30–40 minute) but frequent sessions (ideally at least twice weekly);
- the need for overlearning, with the same material repeated and adopted across sessions;
- the need to communicate session aims and content to other members of the multi-professional team, so they can help consolidate the work;
- the need to remind clients, regularly, of the reasons for meetings, i.e. to address their sexual offending proclivities (it is easy to present interesting and stimulating exercises; it is harder to anchor the purpose of these in the thoughts of our patients – meaning can be lost);
- particularly with this client group, to enable them to take choices, and to respect their individuality;
- to advise, assist and befriend;
- the need to educate and influence the attitudes of staff towards this client group.

It is not inevitable that a sexual offender with learning difficulties will reoffend. Patients with learning difficulties can fall in love, can be confused about their sexuality, have needs for intimacy and tenderness – in other words, have the same range of experience as those caring for them.

STAFF TRAINING AND SUPPORT

Within Special Hospitals and prisons there is an enthusiasm expressed by some staff members for involvement in the treatment of sexual offenders. Of course, this has to be set against attitudes expressed by other staff members which might emphasise punishment rather than treatment, beliefs that sexual offenders cannot be taught to control their behaviour and that those motivated to work with sexual offenders must in themselves be somehow sexually deviant. Such beliefs are not within the sole ownership of any one profession, nor are they restricted to institutions.

Those working in prisons and Special Hospitals represent a hetero-geneous group of individuals, in terms of clinical experience, past training, and opportunities for further training. Some professional groups are more experienced in working with issues pertaining to offending behaviour, and indeed enjoy and promote the status which this affords, in comparison with their less experienced colleagues. Sometimes this leads to some individuals believing their skills to be superior to those of others, for them to overly emphasise dependency and immaturity in their less experienced colleagues and to de-emphasise their own needs for training and development. These dynamics detract from the proper multi-professional training and collabor-ation which are essential in sex offender work.

In both therapist selection and ongoing supervision of case work it will be important for managers of projects to be made aware of practitioners' development needs, their strengths and weaknesses and deficiencies in their knowledge base. This challenges the staff training colleges of our prison service to research and resource the needs of uniformed staff in particular. The onus on each practitioner is to communicate these needs and to remind themselves that true 'professional' practice means operating within the bounds of one's competence.

Each manager in turn has a responsibility to ensure that clear structures and policy operate in relation to sex offender work within institutions, and that the necessary resources are made available for that work to be carried out. Inmates and staff have to be protected from the adverse effects of mismanaged projects. The issue of who should manage projects is, of course, not straightforward. Whilst the governors of prisons or responsible medical officers (consultant grade psychiatrists) in Special Hospitals might assume overall responsibility for the care of individuals, they are most probably not the persons immediately responsible for offering assessment and therapy. The clear communication of therapeutic goals is essential between members of therapeutic teams and also between those teams and team or project managers.

Multi-professional working

Proper multi-professional working within institutions, including compre-hensive sentence or treatment planning, is, as already indicated, hard to achieve. Targets for such can be identified, however. The recommend-ations of an internal task force at Rampton Hospital on patient care planning suggested the following targets for the care planning process:

- there should be one multi-disciplinary treatment plan per patient;
- the planning process should allow for flexibility within the general framework;
- key individuals in the planning process should be identified;
- communication between members of the multi-disciplinary team is essential;
- the patient should be involved in the treatment planning process wherever possible;
- treatment plans should be regularly reviewed by the multi-disciplinary team, the timing of these reviews depending on treatment requirements;
- assessment and treatment should be offered at a time and a place best suited to the patient's needs;
- the process of treatment planning should be easily communicated and should be responsive to current practices;
- the process of treatment planning should encourage the active involvement of all members of the multi-disciplinary team.

The process should foster the responsibilities of different professions working within the team. Frameworks for support are essential at several levels, particularly supervision, consultancy, peer support and external support. All are important for practitioners within institutions at all points in their professional development. This has significant resource implications for the managers of programmes. Programme managers have to make commitments to releasing staff for training and support throughout the lifespan of the project. Other priorities should not cut across the maintenance of established projects.

Support of practitioners should not ignore personal issues. Staff often feel vulnerable when they are subject to the criticism and hostility of those colleagues who are unsympathetic to sex offender work, or to the emotions aroused by the content of the work. Such issues (which are discussed in Chapter 9) are particularly difficult to resolve within institutions that lack an ethos of personal disclosure of uncomfortable emotions or feelings by its workforce. At the present stage in our understanding of 'what works' with sexual offenders, there are more unknowns than knowns. Accordingly, one of the most important skills any practitioner might bring to an institutional treatment programme for perpetrators is that of the applied scientist – an open, questioning and empirical practice base, including a healthy scepticism for much self-reported material. Finally, practitioners need a supportive yet challenging style which motivates the inmate to accept long-term responsibility for their offending.

Experience of training many prison and Special Hospital staff indicates that the content of any training course needs to include models which describe and structure the phenomena of sexual offending, information about the context of offender work (the legal and penal systems; the roles and background of professional groups; management, accountability and policy frameworks; rehabilitation issues, including responsibilities towards schedule one offenders and those proposed for trial leave or parole) and the provision of therapy skills and theories of sex offender treatment.

Individual and group work skills are essential, including co-therapy skills, the skills of functional analysis and those of behavioural counselling and skills training. One of the most basic yet crucial skills of offender work, that of interviewing to obtain information about the inmate's offence, sadly is often the skill most poorly developed in institutional practitioners, and an essential focus of staff training. Feedback from those who have attended training courses emphasises the value in training staff to work in depth with offenders, in training them to understand and manage the phenomena of denial and to understand the phenomena of relapse and recidivism. The opportunity for institutional staff to observe and participate in therapy groups for offenders, run in other institutions and the community, is much valued.

WHAT NEXT

To improve the quality of our interventions with sexual offenders in institutions, we must deal with several issues:

1 We must intervene earlier in the development of offence histories. Considerable thought and attention should be directed at the imprisoned adolescent sexual offender population. We also need to prevent the sexual violation of adolescents in institutional care.
2 Active and offence-focused treatment should be offered to patients and prisoners on reception to institutions. We should avoid the situation where clients are allowed to fantasise for several years about illegal acts whilst awaiting offers of therapy.
3 Staff should be properly supported in their work with offenders. This has obvious implications. Staff should have access to proper and on-going training, supervision and consultancy. They should have the resources, management support and opportunity to conduct this work.
4 In our enthusiasm to become involved in the assessment and treatment of sex offenders we have a responsibility to maintain the integrity of treatments and to protect clients from the abuse and misuse of our technologies.
5 Most importantly we have to adopt a scientific attitude to our work. Research is needed to explore both the process of therapy as well as its effectiveness. Client groups should not be neglected – for example,

those with learning difficulties, female sex offenders, and those from minority ethnic groups. We should not ignore issues such as the efficiency of treatment, the identification of likely responders, nor the contra-indications of intervention. The development of broader data-bases across institutions and the collaboration of prison service and Special Hospital staff in research activity should be encouraged. We have a busy time ahead!

7   Adolescent sexual abusers

Research, assessment and treatment

Dave O'Callaghan and Bobbie Print

Recognition of the overall proportion of sexual assaults committed by young people has stimulated practitioners, both in North America and latterly in the UK, to attempt to develop appropriate services to work with this group. Within the UK a feature of this development has been the range of agencies and disciplines represented in the service provision developed so far. For example, practitioners are involved from child protection, probation, youth justice, child and adolescent psychiatry and forensic services.

The area of work with young people who sexually abuse is, in fact, a pivotal one in which professionals with varying experiences and philosophies are attempting to establish a consistent approach. The danger is the development of competition and elitism, rather than a service benefiting from a complementary range of skills. Organisational imperatives can also mitigate against productive interagency developments. Our aim in this chapter is to consider the research base which can assist in developing a common understanding of the problem and to examine the establishment and operation of a multi-agency programme working with young abusers, and the practical issues raised.

UNDERSTANDING THE SEXUAL BEHAVIOUR OF YOUNG PEOPLE

Defining normal, problematic or abusive sexual behaviours is a major difficulty for professionals with responsibilities for young people. The uncertainty created can make us feel powerless to respond to behaviours that trouble or concern us. Consequently a framework is needed to assist our understanding of abusive incidents and behaviours. Two of the core concepts which should form the basis of such a framework are consent and power.

Consent

Interpersonal sexual behaviour which does not involve mutually consenting participants is abusive. The issue of consent by children is often confused with compliance or cooperation. The definition developed by Adamas and Fay (1984) is particularly useful in clarifying the basic concepts:

> Consent is based on choice. Consent is active not passive. Consent is possible only when there is equal power. Forcing someone to give in is not consent. Going along with something because of wanting to fit in with the group is not consent. . . . If you can't say 'no' comfortably then 'yes' has no meaning. If you are unwilling to accept a 'no' then 'yes' has no meaning.

The elements of consent can be summarised as:

• understanding the proposal;
• knowing the standard (i.e. societal definition/regard) of that behaviour;
• being aware of the possible consequences;
• knowledge that any decision will be respected.

Power

In abusive situations the power of the abuser is used to deny the victim free choice. Some of the principal elements of power differentials in sexual relationships can be summarised as follows:

• age, gender, race and culture;
• physical size/strength;
• significant different levels of cognitive functioning;
• invested authority (e.g. babysitting, school prefect);
• self-image differential;
• arbitrary labels (e.g. such as leader in games).

Applying the above framework of consent and power allows us to define adolescent sexual behaviours in terms of whether they are acceptable/ normal, require limited intervention/further assessment or are clearly abusive and require treatment. The following categorisations are examples of adolescent sexual behaviours adapted from those developed by Ryan and Lane (1991):

Normal behaviours

• explicit sexual discussion amongst peers, use of sexual swear words, obscene jokes;

- interest in erotic material and its use in masturbation;
- expression through sexual innuendo, flirtations and courtship behaviours;
- mutual consenting non-coital sexual behaviour (kissing, fondling, etc.);
- mutual consenting masturbation;
- mutual consenting sexual intercourse.

Behaviours that suggest monitoring, limited responses or assessment

- sexual preoccupation/anxiety;
- use of hard core pornography;
- indiscriminate sexual activity/intercourse;
- twinning of sexuality and aggression;
- sexual graffiti relating to individuals or having disturbing content;
- single occurrences of exposure, peeping, frottage or obscene telephone calls.

Behaviours that suggest assessment/intervention

- compulsive masturbation if chronic or public;
- persistent or aggressive attempts to expose others' genitals;
- chronic use of pornography with sadistic or violent themes;
- sexually explicit conversations with significantly younger children;
- touching another's genitals without permission;
- sexually explicit threats.

Behaviours that require a legal response, assessment and treatment

- persistent obscene telephone calls, voyeurism, exhibitionism or frottage;
- sexual contact with significantly younger children;
- forced sexual assault and rape;
- inflicting genital injury;
- sexual contact with animals.

Sgroi's assessment methodology (1989) underlines the developmental perspective and highlights the use of secrecy:

> does the sexual behaviour initiated by a child fit into anticipated developmental norms with regard to ages of the participants, patterns of activity and sexual behaviours . . . Did the child who initiated the sexual behaviour do so openly or furtively? With concern about discovery or disregard for being detected? Were other participants bribed or threatened? What did the victim think would happen if she or he told others?

Reported rates of incidence

An important stimulus to the development of treatment programmes directed at adolescent sex abusers has been the growing recognition that they account for a sizeable proportion of reported sexual victimisation.

More than a decade ago Finkelhor's (1979) survey of 796 female college students reported that a third of those who disclosed victimisation identified their abuser as aged between 10 and 19 years at the time of the abuse. Havgaard and Tilley (1988), in surveying 1,000 undergraduates found that 42 per cent reported experiencing a sexual encounter during childhood with a child or young person. Fromuth *et al.* (1991) surveyed 582 college males and found 3 per cent reported having abused one or more children (aged 3–12 years) when they were 16–17 years of age.

One of the few UK non-clinical samples is that of 1,244 16 to 21-year-olds surveyed by Kelly *et al.* (1991). Of those respondents who reported an abusive history or experience, 27 per cent of perpetrators were identified as aged 13–17 years of age and 1 per cent aged 12 years or less at the time of assault.

Whilst such 'community-based' surveys offer some confirmation that the pattern of adolescent sexual abuse identified in clinical populations reflects realistic rates, it is via studies of identified abusive incidents that the significance of adolescents as abusers has been established. Dube and Herbert (1988) reviewed 511 cases of victimised children aged less than 12: 26 per cent of identified abusers were aged less than 15; 22 per cent between 15 and 20 and 19 per cent between 20 and 30 years of age. A study by Gomes-Schwartz *et al.* (1990) of 156 children found adolescents identified as the abuser in one-third of cases. Davies and Leitenberg's (1987) review of research found adolescents to be abusers in 30–50 per cent of cases.

To date the vast majority of research available has come from North America, and questions may arise as to its relevance in the UK. Although available statistics are limited in this country, those we have access to appear to show a similar pattern of adolescent sexual offending to that demonstrated by the North American studies. Criminal statistics (Home Office, 1990b) covering offences reported during 1989 show that out of the 10,729 individuals found guilty or cautioned for sexual offences, one-third were aged 20 years or younger:

> 17–20 years . . . . 20 per cent (n. 2,146)
> 14–16 years . . . . 9 per cent (n. 965)
> 10–13 years . . . . 3 per cent (n. 322)

The most extensive UK research project to date has been the Northern Ireland study (Northern Ireland Research Team, 1991), which examined

408 cases of child sex abuse. The study found that in 36.1 per cent of cases the abuser was an adolescent. In 20.5 per cent of cases the abuser was aged 16 years or less.

WHO IS VICTIMISED?

Age

The Northern Ireland study (ibid.) identified a statistically significant relationship between the age of the abuser and that of the victim. Of the group of children victimised by 16-year-olds, half were aged under 9 years and two-thirds under 12.

That victims of adolescent abusers are predominantly in the younger age group is supported by North American research. Fehrenbach's (1983) study found that the median age of victims of adolescent abusers was 6 years. Later Fehrenbach *et al.* (1986) found 60 per cent of victims to be aged less than 12 years. Becker and Kaplan's (1988) study of adolescent sex offenders found 60 per cent of victims to be aged less than 8 years. Farrel and O'Brien's (1988) survey of 731 cases of child sexual assault found that the average victim's age was between 5 and 7 years and the median age of the offender was 14. Ryan and Lane's (ibid.) review of the data collected by the National Adolescent Perpetrator Network found that in only 15 per cent of cases was the victim of sexual assault a peer or older.

Gender

Kahn and Lafond's (1988) study found 30 per cent of adolescent sex offenders victimised both males and females; 20 per cent victimised males only and 40 per cent females only. In Becker and Stein's (1991) study, 65 per cent of victims were female, while Fromuth *et al.* (1991) reported that 67 per cent of victims were female. Becker and Stein additionally discovered that those adolescents who disclosed a personal history of sexual abuse appeared equally as likely to abuse males (49 per cent) as females (51 per cent).

Awad and Saunders' (1991) study contrasts juvenile 'sexual assaulters' with juvenile 'child molesters' (those with victims four or more years younger) and juvenile non-sex offenders. Whilst none of the sample of sexual assaulters was identified as victimising males, 41 per cent of the child molester group were. This latter group also presented with a personal history of sexual victimisation at a significantly higher rate than the assaulter or delinquent groups. This study also found that the child molester victims were more likely to have been repeatedly abused. Kahn and

Chambers' (1991) study of 221 adolescent sex offenders found that of those offenders with a single victim, the gender split of victims was 26 per cent male and 74 per cent female, whereas the split was 56 per cent male and 44 per cent female for those offenders who targeted three or more victims.

These studies reflect Becker *et al.*'s (1989) finding that abusers identified as victimised (primarily by males) presented with a more deviant sexual arousal to prepubescent males on psycho-physiological testing. Further evidence of this pattern is shown in O'Brien's (1991) study showing that of those adolescent offenders abused by males, nearly 70 per cent of their subsequent victims were male. In Hunter's (1991) sample of 52 sexual abuse victims, 68 per cent of the males were assaulted by an adolescent, in comparison to 14 per cent of the females victimised.

Relationships

Research and clinical experience indicate that access to victims plays a central role in the pattern of adolescent sexual abuse. Adolescents are less mobile and less likely to have an adult abuser's skills in targeting victims. Kahn and Lafond's (1988) study found that 95 per cent of adolescent abusers knew their victims and the most common link was a sibling or a child for whom the adolescent was babysitting – a finding supported by Margolin's (1993) study of abuse by care-givers, in which adolescents were heavily represented in abuse committed by babysitters. In a further study of adolescent abusers (Kahn and Chambers, 1991) 31 per cent of victims were known to the abuser but of a different household, and 28 per cent were a blood-related sibling.

One-third of offences (38.7 per cent) in the National Adolescent Perpetrator Network sample (Ryan and Lane, 1991) were found to be against members of the same household. Pierce and Pierce (1990), reviewing 43 adolescent intra-familial offenders, found the sibling relationship predominant: 20 per cent of victims were natural, step- or adoptive sisters; 19 per cent were foster sisters; 16 per cent were foster brothers; 5 per cent were natural brothers.

A total of 67 per cent of Wiehe's (1990) study of 150 adults who reported childhood experiences of sibling abuse identified themselves as sexually abused. Over half of these reported that the sexual abuse was accompanied by a degree of physical and or emotional abuse.

In a substantive comparative evaluation by O'Brien (1991) of intra- and extra-familial adolescent abusers, he identifies the former as being:

• more likely to engage in penetrative intercourse;

- more likely to assault more than one child;
- having a history of abusing that tended to go undiscovered for longer periods.

Logically one can assume these findings reflect the intra-familial abuser's greater access to victims, resulting in an ability to 'groom' and desensitise victims to more intrusive sexual contact and to exercise control over victims' ability to disclose. It is perhaps particularly important to emphasise the care context as providing adolescents' access to vulnerable children. A study of abuse in out-of-home placements, by Rosenthal *et al.* (1991), identified 37 per cent of sexual assaults as perpetrated either by a fellow residential care resident (16 per cent) or foster sibling (21 per cent).

CHARACTERISTICS OF THE ADOLESCENT SEXUAL ABUSER

Comparison with the wider delinquent population

A number of studies have attempted to differentiate the adolescent sex offender from the wider group of youths engaged in criminal behaviours. These generally conclude there are minimal statistically significant differences between the two groups (Smith, 1988; McCraw and Pegg-McNab, 1989).

If any difference does emerge, it is that adolescent sexual abusers are found to be otherwise less delinquent. Becker and Kaplan (1988) found that most of the adolescent sex offenders in their study had experienced no previous contact with the criminal justice system. Fagan and Wexler (1988) studied a group of 34 sex offenders out of a total of 242 juvenile offenders. They found the sex offender group were more likely to be living in households with natural parents, were less likely to have committed violent (non-sexual) offences and had lower self-reported rates of substance abuse or other delinquent activities. This is echoed in Awad and Saunders' (1991) study, where the 'sexual assaulters' group were less likely than the delinquents to have a history of alcohol abuse or of drug abuse, and in Bagley's (1992) comparative survey, where the sexually abusive group were significantly less likely than the non-sex offenders to engage in property offences or non-sexual assaults. These findings are supported by our own study in Greater Manchester, where we have compared the characteristics of 50 adolescent male sex offenders with a group of 28 adolescents with convictions for non-sexual offences. The adolescent sex offenders' involvement in a range of 'delinquent' behaviours, including drug abuse, theft, criminal damage, car theft and violence, was significantly less than that of the non-sex offender group.

Social development

Research frequently identifies social skills deficits as a recurrent and significant feature of the adolescent sexual abuser's social presentation (Fehrenbach *et al.*, 1986; Saunders and Awad, 1988; Fagan and Wexler, 1988). Most commonly noted is an inability to make and sustain meaningful peer group friendships, and difficulties in assertion and anger control. In the Awad and Saunders (1991) study, two-thirds of the child molesters group were identified as socially isolated, compared with one-third of the adult assaulters group. Bagley (1992) found his sexually abusive group of adolescents displayed more hyperactivity, anxiety, depression, poor self-concept and suicidal ideas or behaviour than the group who had committed non-sexual offences.

Our own Manchester study (Beckett *et al.*, in preparation) has similar findings, with adolescent sexual abusers exhibiting relatively high degrees of withdrawal and social anxiety compared to those involved in non-sex offences. Approximately twice as many sexual abusers as non-sex offenders reported that they had been bullied in school and many felt that they had few friends or social contacts. This social isolation also impacted on the adolescent's 'dating' behaviour and we found that only 50 per cent of the sexual abusers in the Manchester study had a number of girlfriends, compared to 81 per cent of the non-sex offenders. Only 26 per cent had experienced regular sexual intercourse with a peer (non-abusive), compared to 59 per cent of the non-sex offending group, and 32 per cent of the sexual abusers believed that they were less successful with girls than their peers, compared to 19 per cent of the non-sex offenders.

Educational/academic development

Studies generally note that the adolescent sexual abuser is likely to struggle with the educational system, often presenting as a low achiever or having learning difficulties (Fehrenbach *et al.*, 1986; Saunders and Awad, 1988). Kahn and Chambers (1991) found half their sample had histories of disruptive behaviour at school; one-third had a history of truancy and 39 per cent were considered learning disabled. Our study (op. cit.) has highlighted that whilst half the sexual abusers perceived themselves as having learning difficulties, as compared to 19 per cent of non-sex offenders, their general intelligence level was very similar to the non-sex offender group.

Experiences of prior victimisation

As literature describing clinical populations of adolescent sexual abusers has increased, awareness of many abusers' experiences of victimisation has grown. Models of adolescent sexual abuse have now been developed which include prior victimisation as a core factor in the development of abusive behaviour (Ryan *et al.*, 1987). Evidence on the percentage of young abusers who have themselves been victims of sexual abuse is variable. Becker *et al.* (1988) and Becker and Stein (1991) have been researching this issue, amongst others, for some years and report that an average of almost 30 per cent of young abusers disclose prior abuse. Sefarbi (1990) reported 25 per cent; Awad and Saunders' (1991) child molester group 21 per cent; O'Brien (1991) reported 40 per cent, Pierce and Pierce (1990) found 48 per cent; Kahn and Lafond's (1988) large sample (350) contained a high percentage, approaching 60 per cent, who reported prior victimisation. Intriguingly, two similar studies arrived at very different conclusions: both Bagley (1992) and Benoit and Kennedy (1992) undertook comparative research on groups of sexual and non-sexual offenders. Bagley found a higher statistical proportion of the sexually abusive group had experienced prior sexual victimisation, whilst the latter study found no statistical difference between the two groups.

Overall whilst research and practice does appear to demonstrate that experience of sexual victimisation is a significant factor in the development of sexually abusive behaviours, Benoit and Kennedy's (ibid.) comment does appear to have a general relevance: 'This study, which does not purport to prove the null hypothesis, suggests that the relationship between being a victim of certain types of abuse and subsequent offending is not direct; other factors must be in operation.'

Characteristics of families

Interest has grown as to whether the families of adolescent sexual abusers display any common characteristics. Smith and Israel (1987) examined the families of 25 adolescent intra-familial abusers and identified a discernible pattern of internal family dynamics:

- distant, inaccessible parents;
- parents who stimulated a sexual climate in their home;
- family history of maintaining secrets.

The data base of the National Adolescent Perpetrator Network (1988) holds information on over 1,000 adolescent sex offenders and reports the following statistics: parental loss in 57 per cent of cases; spouse abuse in 28 per cent; substance abuse in 27 per cent of mothers and 43 per cent of fathers. Only 28 per cent of juveniles were living with both parents at the time of the offence. The vast majority of families were evaluated as 'below average', 'inappropriate' or 'dysfunctional'. Bagley's study (1992) found that young abusers were likely to be within intact families, but that these families exhibited high levels of marital tension, instability and mental illness.

In the Manchester study (Beckett *et al.*, in preparation), 38 per cent of the sexual abusers lived with stepfathers and 12 per cent reported that their parents had separated because of violence in the marital relationship. Eighteen per cent reported that their father had served a term of imprisonment (non-sex offences), compared with 4 per cent of the non-sex offender group. Forty-one per cent of the sexual abusers reported that their siblings were better treated by their parents. During treatment, all of the young abusers we have worked with have reported feeling isolated within their family.

Kaplan *et al.* (1988) conducted structured interviews with 27 parents of adolescent intra-familial sexual abusers. Only two had received hospital treatment for mental health problems. Some 96 per cent had no arrest record for non-sexual crimes, whilst 9.1 per cent had at least one arrest for a sexual crime. Twenty-seven per cent disclosed a prior experience of physical abuse and 30 per cent of sexual abuse. Only half were able to fully acknowledge their sons' abusive behaviours. The majority had undertaken no sex education with their children. In Michael O'Brien's (1991) study comparing intra- and extra-familial adolescent abusers, 36 per cent of mothers and 10 per cent of fathers in the intra-familial sample disclosed an experience of sexual victimisation. This differed from the extra-familial sample, where the figures were 9 per cent and 5.5 per cent respectively. Kahn and Lafond, (1988) identified a known abuser, other than the adolescent, in the household or family in half the cases they surveyed. A total of one-third identified a family member as abused by someone other than the adolescent referred. This finding was replicated in research by Lankester and Meyer (1986), who studied 153 adolescent sex offenders and reported that 64 per cent of family members had been either physically or sexually abused as children.

Sefarbi (1990) evaluated the families of two groups of adolescent sexual abusers: those admitting and those denying the offence. She identified the deniers' families as 'disengaged', noting a psychological or actual (physical) abandonment. In contrast, the admitters were identified as living within 'enmeshed' families, isolated from social contacts and used in a partnership role by parents either for emotional support or practical help such as babysitting.

CURRENT TREATMENT PROGRAMMES

Early treatment is important, not only to prevent further offending but because the prognosis is considered better with adolescents who have not yet developed ingrained patterns of behaviour, attitudes or belief systems. There is an additional advantage in working with young people in that professional, family and community support networks are often more readily available to them than to adults.

In recent years there has been a dramatic growth in the number of treatment facilities for adolescent abusers in the United States. Knopp *et al.* (1992) have tracked this development and reports that the number of programmes more than doubled in the period 1986 to 1992, from 346 to 755.

As with adult abusers, there is a consensus of opinion amongst those working in the field, that treatment for adolescents who sexually abuse others aims to protect the community by helping the abusers to control their behaviour. The underlying philosophies of many of the programmes are related to those seen in adult sex offenders programmes. There is acceptance that adolescent sex abusers have developed a dysfunctional behaviour which is not generally mitigated by time alone. The deviant behaviours and thinking processes of the abusers originate from negative experiences, such as various forms of abuse in childhood, which lead to the abuser developing deep needs for power, acceptance and aggression which they meet through abusive sexual behaviour. The secrecy, perceived sense of power, arousal and masturbation to deviant fantasies may then serve to reinforce the abusive behaviour to the extent that it becomes compulsive.

Although this theoretical concept has formed the basis of much of the work undertaken with adolescents who sexually abuse others, there are still many unanswered questions regarding the development and maintenance of sexually abusive behaviour. For example, there are as yet no clear indications as to what specific characteristics, experiences or circumstances are the most significant in the development of sexually abusive behaviour; which adolescents are most likely to reabuse, or what issues are most effective to address in treatment.

North American treatment programmes that have been developed reflect this lack of specific knowledge in their variation of content and methods. Many programmes attempt to address a wide range of issues which are believed to cause and maintain an adolescent's abusive behaviour. Over 80 per cent of respondents in Knopp *et al.*'s survey (1992) describe their programmes as based on behavioural-cognitive, psycho-social-educational or relapse prevention models. Other programmes focus on the one or two specific issues which they believe may be the most effective in preventing further offending. For details of some North American adolescent programmes, see Becker *et al.* (1988), Ryan *et al.* (1987), Knopp *et al.* (1992), Ross (1990), Smets and Cebula (1987).

THE GREATER MANCHESTER ADOLESCENT PROGRAMME (G-MAP)

The G-MAP is a multi-agency initiative which was established in 1988 by staff from social services, probation, NSPCC, and the health service. The project consists of three elements – assessment, treatment and research – and offers a service to young people, between the ages of 13 and 18 years, who sexually abuse others. Whilst assessments are undertaken with young people of either gender, the group treatment programme the project runs is for males only as the numbers of identified female adolescent abusers have, as yet, not been sufficient to warrant a group treatment response.

The overriding goal of the G-MAP programme is to protect society from further sexual assaults by attempting to identify the needs of young people who sexually abuse others and to provide therapeutic services to those individuals and families where it is appropriate. The programme has developed an eclectic methodology based largely on humanistic, client-centred and cognitive restructuring therapies. The aim of the work is to help the adolescents recognise, understand and accept responsibility for their abusive behaviour and to develop more appropriate, non-harmful ways of coping with their experiences and situations.

Our approach is to provide a safe environment for the young people in which to reflect on their behaviour, beliefs and attitudes and to support and encourage individual change through the development of knowledge, understanding and insight, improving self-esteem and empathy, and the acquisition of new skills and development of positive support networks. In broad terms this is achieved by the use of firm boundaries, education, group support and mirroring, self-exploration, new skill development and rehearsal, constructive challenge and peer pressure and positive recognition of individual worth and progress.

In addition to group therapy, most programme participants will be involved in individual therapy sessions and in many cases families and/or carers will be involved in therapeutic work.

A model of the G-MAP programme is shown in figure 7.1.

Referrals

Our referral process requires the referrer to provide core information on the following areas:

- the young person's own history and present circumstances;
- family details, history and attitudes – for example, their view of their child's need for treatment;
- precise and detailed information on the young person's assault behaviour;

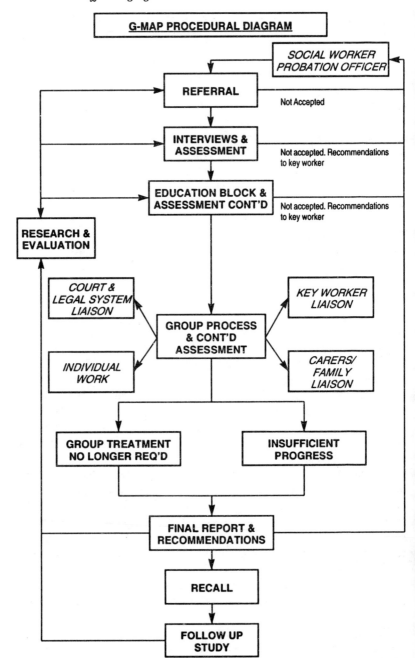

Figure 7.1 Model of the G-MAP programme

- system response, for example, information on any joint police–social services investigation, child protection conference, legal action taken or pending, etc.

Often issues are raised at referral stage that require a response from project staff – for example, where there has been a clear failure to follow child protection procedures, or where the abuser and victim, inappropriately, continue to live in the same household. Staff developing projects should also consider what statistical information may be useful to them in terms of research, project evaluation, responses to management, and elicit such information in referrals.

Assessment

The assessment procedure is considered to have therapeutic value in itself, and although an assessment phase is identified at the start of the programme, the assessment process is considered an integral part of treatment.

The aims of the initial assessment are to determine:

- whether further professional intervention is required;
- whether the abuser is safe enough to remain in the community for treatment;
- whether he/she is motivated to engage in treatment;
- whether he/she is likely to respond to treatment;
- what type of treatment is most suitable;
- what treatment resources are available to him/her.

It is important not to underestimate the risks of further abuse when working with sexual abusers, and to identify those who are not suitable for community-based programmes. In many instances treatment-providers are likely to be under pressure to accept all who are referred, either because alternative treatment facilities are scarce or because referrals are infrequent and those running the programme are keen to increase their numbers. There are several dangers in succumbing to these pressures. Accepting unsuitable referrals into treatment is likely to result in increasing the risk to potential victims, unsatisfactory results which discredit the programme, other group members being inhibited and unsettled, and inappropriate messages being given to the abuser concerned, who may well consider that he has 'beaten the system'.

The identification of an individual's treatment needs and risk of re-offending are based on the assessment of his support network, beliefs, thoughts and behaviour, strengths and weaknesses, past experiences, skills and deficits. The assessment approach developed by G-MAP contains a number of discrete phases:

Information gathering

In addition to the completed referral form, information is also collected from a structured interview with parents or carers, victim and abuser depositions or statements, any previous assessments, previous court reports, case conference minutes, relevant medical reports, school reports and any other relevant source.

Individual interviews

Kaplan *et al.* (1991) have produced evidence which suggests that a male and female interviewer working together are most effective for initial interviews with adolescent sexual abusers. In the light of this, G-MAP conducts a series of three semi-structured interviews using a male and a female worker in each case.

The initial interview is used to explore with the adolescent his/her personal history, family experiences, social behaviours and sexual development. The first interview is used as a forum to establish some rapport with the young person. The interviewers introduce themselves and give their understanding for the young person's referral to the programme. The nature and aims of the assessment are explained, together with the consequences of the adolescent's cooperation or non-cooperation in completing the process. Emphasis is given to the need for honesty during the assessment and acknowledgement is given that some parts might be embarrassing or painful for him/her. By then focusing on personal history details it is unlikely that the adolescent will feel the need to deny or minimise his/her abusive behaviour. Most participants feel reasonably comfortable in answering questions about their history and in this way it is possible that they will begin to relax and allow some positive rapport to be established.

The establishment of this rapport is an important foundation for the second interview when adolescents are asked to give details of the assault/s they have committed, the antecedents to the assault/s, any planning or rehearsal, use of coercion, their feelings and behaviour before the abuse and afterwards, together with their understanding of the effects on victims. The adolescents are questioned about who they have told about the abusive behaviour and how honest they have been.

The interview is designed to be a motivational interview, where an adolescent is encouraged to answer questions in as much detail as possible. Any distortions in his/her views of what happened or why are not forcefully challenged at this stage, as the purpose of the interview is to elicit as much detail as possible regarding the young person's thinking. This is not to say, however, that unacceptable attitudes, denial or dishonesty are not responded to by the interviewer. It is important that concern about such matters is raised at the end of the interview, to avoid any possibility of perceived collusion by the abuser.

Most adolescents find the interview uncomfortable, and the skill of the interviewer is to balance this discomfort with an atmosphere that allows the offender to provide details of his/her thoughts, feelings and behaviours which underpin the abusive behaviour. Questions are asked in a way that elicits the fine detail of events leading up to, during and after the last assault. Other incidents of abusive behaviour are then examined to see how they differed to the last assault. The adolescent is encouraged to use this opportunity to further shed feelings of anxiety and guilt and to assist the production of an accurate assessment by sharing details of any previously undisclosed abusive behaviour.

It is useful to adopt a matter-of-fact manner, using open-ended and assumptive questions. When combined with a positive reinforcement of apparent honesty and disclosure by the abuser, these motivational interviewing techniques have proved effective in eliciting a significant level of information.

The final interview is used to examine with the young person their views and attitudes about the abuse, and other related issues. Details of the adolescent's sexual fantasies, sexual knowledge and experiences are explored and his/her views on the advantages and disadvantages of attending a treatment programme are elicited.

Psychological testing

A range of pen and paper tests are used, some of which are generally available, for example the Jesness Inventory (Jesness, 1962) which examines attitudes and beliefs, and the Multiphasic Sex Inventory Juvenile Form (Nichols and Molinder, 1984), which examines sexual behaviour, cognitions and treatment attitudes. Other questionnaires have been developed specifically for the programme, such as a victim empathy scale and a self-esteem inventory. The test results are evaluated by a psychologist and used primarily for research purposes. As many of the tests used have not yet been standardised in this country, the information they provide is only used to enhance the information gained in other ways.

Initial assessment

An initial assessment of each adolescent is carried out at this stage. The information gathered is used to consider:

1 **The need for further professional intervention** For some young people, it may be decided that the behaviour they engaged in was of an experimental nature which did not result in significant trauma for the victim. Such cases would include circumstances where the young person had fully cooperated with the assessment process, had not physically or aggressively coerced the victim, had not planned the abuse, had ceased the abuse upon objection from the victim, had not engaged in any penetrative assault, had not used threats to silence the victim, had not maintained denial when confronted, had no significant inappropriate fantasies, and who had no personal or family history that raised concerns. In these cases it may be that involvement in the assessment process and examination of their behaviour and its consequences is sufficient to ensure that the young person is unlikely to commit further abuse.

   In other cases, whilst a further professional response is identified as necessary, it may not be appropriate for the individual to attend a long-term group treatment programme. For example, some adolescents may be better suited to individual therapy and others may be identified as only requiring a short, intensive education input. In such cases a recommendation is made regarding the needs of the individual and appropriate resources identified wherever possible.

2 **Level of denial** In order to be accepted into the G-MAP treatment programme, an adolescent must acknowledge that he committed the abuse for which he has been referred. At this stage it is accepted that adolescents who have sexually abused others are likely to be rationalising, minimising or projecting blame onto others. Abusers who totally deny that they committed the offence, or those who do not accept any measure of responsibility, are unlikely to be considered for inclusion in the programme.

3 **Assessment of risk** Assessment of risk is a complex process which relies on an informed analysis of many factors elicited during the assessment process. The risk assessment is fundamental to the formulation of recommendations regarding treatment provision, prosecution, contact with children, and so on. Additionally, not all adolescents who have sexually abused others will be suitable for treatment in the community. Some will be assessed as being at high risk of reoffending and will require treatment in a residential or custodial setting. In broad terms, contra-indications of suitability for treatment in the community include:

— a history of serious physical violence and/or violent or sadistic fantasies;
— a long history of truancy or absconding;
— reoffences following completion of previous appropriate treatment programmes;
— other indications of very poor impulse control, for example frequent aggressive outbursts;
— serious, ongoing substance misuse;
— failure to cooperate with the assessment process.

Adolescents who habitually misuse substances are not admitted to the programme. Their key workers are advised that the offender may be re-referred to the programme once their misuse is under control.

4 **Motivation**   The legal status of the abuser, together with his reasons for wishing to attend the programme, are considered. Experience and the results of pre-group testing during assessment in the Manchester programme have shown that adolescents are rarely, if ever, initially self-motivated to attend for treatment and most will not fully engage or remain in treatment unless they are concerned about the consequences of not doing so. The assessment identifies the minimum mandate which is considered necessary to protect the public and to ensure the young person receives the response he/she requires. Recommendations may therefore include: no further legal action, police caution, civil action under the Children Act 1989, or criminal prosecution. In addition, other recommendations may be made regarding placements, restricted contact with children, curfew, etc.

Among the positive motivational indicators for involvement in the G-MAP programme are:

— a legal mandate to attend for treatment;
— other significant consequences of not receiving treatment, e.g. non-return to family;
— a positive attitude towards treatment in the abuser's family and those with whom he lives;
— a genuine desire to change.

The adolescent's school and employment record are also explored to establish whether they have demonstrated significant patterns of disrupted attendance or lack of commitment.

Unless it is thought that there are significant identifiable consequences for an abuser who drops out or is excluded from the treatment, he is unlikely to be accepted onto the G-MAP programme. Our experience leads us to concur with the National Task Force Report

(NAPN, 1988) which states: 'Treatment orders which expire regardless of offenders' participation or success in treatment are a threat to community safety as well as the credibility of all treatment.'

5 **Social and intellectual skills** The assessment of any adolescents who have demonstrated such severe social or learning skill deficits that it seems unlikely that they will be able to benefit from a group programme will be completed at this stage and recommendations made regarding alternative treatment modalities. This would include those whose behaviour is so extreme that they would not be accepted by other group members, and abusers who are diagnosed as psychotic. Adolescents with less serious anti-social traits or learning difficulties are not necessarily excluded at this stage, but their performance in the following three-day education block will be closely monitored to further evaluate their potential to benefit from the programme. It is not uncommon for the peer pressure, support and challenge arising in group to bring about positive changes in these areas.

Three-day education block

Adolescents considered suitable for the G-MAP group treatment programme are included in the next stage of assessment and are involved in a three-day group education programme. The involvement in an intense brief programme with other sexual abusers allows a fuller assessment of the adolescent's beliefs, behaviours, intellectual abilities and social skills.

The aims of the three-day block are:

- to complete the pre-group assessment;
- to provide information about the problem of sexually assaultive behaviour, why adolescents commit sex assaults, why denial is so common and what the effects on victims are;
- to provide the participants with information regarding the aims, rules and format of the group;
- to help them to begin to identify issues they need to address;
- to assess their competence in a group setting.

The group leaders run a series of sessions during the programme. The methods include didactic teaching, questionnaires, learning exercises, videotaped programmes and discussion. The programme content consists of:

- attitudes towards sex, sexual deviance and sexuality;
- consequences of sexually abusive behaviour;
- the psychology of the those who sexually abuse others;
- the treatment group, expectations and rules.

The information gathered during the complete assessment phase is collated and used to assess suitability for programme admission and to formulate specific treatment goals for each participant.

Offenders considered unsuitable for the G-MAP treatment group are identified and an assessment report is completed which includes recommendations regarding alternative options. In many cases those who are excluded from the programme at this stage are invited to re-apply at a future date.

The treatment group

Groupwork is the primary therapeutic approach of G-MAP and is acknowledged as the preferred modality by most professionals engaged in working with adolescent sexual abusers (Ryan and Lane, 1991; Steen and Monnette, 1989). Knopp *et al.*'s (1992) survey found that groupwork was the preferred method of working with young abusers in 86 per cent of service providers. Only 2 per cent responded that they used individual treatment alone by choice. Groupwork provides the adolescent with a safe environment in which to explore his sexual behaviour, thoughts and feelings. Social skills and improved self-esteem are often developed through group empathy, support and role-modelling, and peer pressure is very effective in breaking down denial and minimisation.

G-MAP operates an open-ended, weekly group which is part of a rolling programme with an intake twice a year. Each participant's progress is reviewed and most will remain in programme for a minimum of one year. Individual work is undertaken, concurrently, by key workers after discussion with group leaders. Group members are also required to complete homework tasks in their own time.

Group rules

Contrary to most groupwork methods where participants are encouraged to participate in group decision making, to determine the group's agenda and group rules or even to take control of the group, it is important in groups for adolescent sexual abusers that the group leaders assume control. Sexual abusers have engaged in behaviour which has involved exerting power over their victims in order to gratify their own needs, so it is important that they should not be allowed to exert inappropriate power in the group. Group leaders have a key role in demonstrating the appropriate use of authority and in setting clear boundaries in the group. Group rules are established from the outset of an individual's participation and form the firm boundary within which support and therapy are offered.

The G-MAP group rules form part of a written service agreement and include:

Participants must refrain from sexually abusive behaviour. Breach of this rule will result in exclusion from the programme.
Participants are expected to be honest in group.
Participants are expected to participate fully in all sessions.
Participants are expected to attend every session. Absence is only allowed in exceptional circumstances. A total of three missed sessions without satisfactory reason will result in exclusion from the programme. Group sessions will start promptly. Participants who are late will not be admitted to the session and counted as absent.
Limited confidentiality is offered to group members. They are informed from the outset that any information gathered during the group or outside of the group can be exchanged with key workers, families or any others it is considered should know.

Group members must, however, maintain confidentiality in relation to each other. They must not discuss the membership of the group or information regarding other members outside of the group. Breach of this confidentiality rule results in exclusion from the group.
Group members are not allowed to associate with each other outside of the group. They must return directly to their place of residence following group sessions and report to a named person upon their return.
All homework assignments must be completed on time. Those who attend group sessions without homework completed will be excluded from the session in the absence of acceptable reasons.

Other rules cover behaviour in and out of the group and include expectations regarding mutual support and compliance with group leaders, the avoidance of verbal or physical aggression, ridicule or intimidation. Group members are also prohibited from using the last names of their victims in order to reduce the risk of victims being identified by other group participants.

If a participant is excluded from the group for a breach of the rules, or because he is not making progress, a final report is completed which identifies progress made and further treatment that is required together with recommendations regarding the consequences of exclusion.

Service agreements

The written service agreement requires the signature of the adolescent who is to attend group, his parents/carers and a representative of the referring agency. Areas covered in the agreement are:

- confidentiality;
- attendance;
- expectations relating to behaviour in group;
- behaviour outside group;
- programme goals;
- expectations of referring agency;
- consequences for young person of exclusion from the programme.

Group leadership

Each group session is co-led by male and female group leaders and observed by a third team member. The task of the group leaders is to structure the content and direction of the group and to manage the group process. This is most effectively achieved by the assignment of different roles to the two group leaders so that one takes responsibility for leading and directing the content of the session, or part of the session, whilst the second monitors the process issues within the group and addresses these when necessary. The observer's role is to record the session and to provide feedback to the group leaders during debriefing. Recording of group sessions is done by use of a form that has been developed to enable each group member's progress to be scored and tracked. Feedback to the group members on their identified progress is provided regularly and participants are invited to comment on or question the scoring.

The group leaders aim to appropriately empower adolescents by helping them to recognise that they can control their own behaviour. This aim is promoted by challenging distorted thoughts and beliefs, providing group members with information about their abusive behaviour, rehearsing new behaviours and attitudes, helping them gain confidence in controlling this behaviour, and improving self-esteem and by showing respect for the progress individuals make in treatment. Most adolescent boys are not used to operating with each other in such a manner and it therefore requires the group leaders to ensure that the appropriate atmosphere is created by carefully monitoring, role-modelling and rewarding positive behaviour.

It is important that the group members feel safe in the group, if honesty is to be established. Individuals are unlikely to feel safe if they believe that the group leaders dislike or are disgusted by them. Leaders must therefore demonstrate that they can have positive regard and respect for an individual whilst they reject the abusive behaviour he has exhibited. Participants must feel that they are supported and cared for if they are to gain the confidence to change, although it is also essential in a group of this nature that denial, inappropriate attitudes and dishonesty are challenged and confronted, in order to promote change.

To achieve the appropriate balance it is important for group leaders to be able to act as effective role models. Group leadership demands the ability to confront in a firm but supportive manner, so that the adolescent feels sufficiently uncomfortable to want to change but is able to recognise that the confrontation is not a personal attack. Being able to feel anger for an individual's behaviour whilst maintaining a degree of empathy for the individual himself is an important personal skill for group leaders to develop. It is equally important that leaders do not collude with an individual's denial, cognitive distortions or sexist attitudes. For example, abusers who present as very 'victim-like' or as easily distressed must not be permitted to avoid issues or confrontation. Distorted thoughts and beliefs should be challenged assertively, calmly, logically and in depth.

Leaders must also ensure that they avoid presenting stereotypical gender roles. It would be pointless to confront sexist attitudes towards males and females amongst the group members if the group leaders were modelling inappropriate behaviour themselves.

The emotional and behavioural demands on group leaders are considerable and can only be met if they are well prepared as a team and have the opportunity to share with and support each other. Debriefing after each group session and regular team building are essential aspects of the team's functioning. For individual members in the team to develop the skills and confidence to operate effectively as a group leader it is important that the team members establish a high degree of trust, honesty and awareness.

Group dynamics

Group leaders have the essential task of monitoring group dynamics. Inevitably groups will naturally progress through a number of phases, including the forming, norming, storming, performing and mourning phases described by Tuckman (1965). Whilst it is important that a group is supported through these stages by the leaders, it is also essential that inappropriate attempts to gain power within the group are controlled and addressed. For example, on one occasion in group it became clear that a participant was being isolated and ridiculed by other group members. This issue was addressed by use of a group sculpt and role play. Group members were helped to recognise their misuse of power and the effects of this on the participant who was being isolated, and the behaviour diminished.

It is also important that group leaders do not allow the group to establish avoidance strategies. Participants may quickly learn that if, for example, they become distressed, angry or withdrawn when certain issues are raised, they can avoid having to deal with them. If problem behaviours have become apparent in group, we have tended to note them as issues and to focus on them in a later session. The use of exercises such as asking each participant to identify ways in which he could sabotage the group and how others might attempt to do the same have proved successful in confronting such behaviours, so that avoidance activities recede.

The phases of change outlined in Chapter 5 of this book, relating to the use of group work with adult sexual abusers, are also applicable to adolescents. The value of a rolling programme is that in many instances established group participants will also identify the particular phase an individual is at and will be able to feed this back to him. For example, those who have been in the group for some time are likely to confront denial in new members very effectively. They may also advise other members that they once held similar beliefs or attitudes and explain what enabled them to move on. An established group that is running well relies heavily on group members facilitating, challenging and supporting each other through change. An open-ended group that has acquired these skills is likely to retain them, irrespective of members joining and leaving, as long as such transitions are carefully planned.

Content issues

Eclectic treatment methods which address cognitive, emotional and behavioural components are employed in presenting the programme content. Due to the complexity and extent of the issues that need to be included in a comprehensive treatment programme, it is necessary to focus on particular themes for a number of sessions. Whilst these themes generally follow the cycle of offending (Ryan and Lane, 1991) they are not precise categories and many issues overlap. The programme content is cyclic, and themes will be addressed in a variety of ways on a number of occasions. In this way an individual can remain in treatment until he has achieved all of his target goals. If he does not make sufficient progress when an issue is addressed on one occasion, he will remain in group until the issue comes round again, when his progress will be re-evaluated.

Issues that are repeatedly addressed in sessions are group dynamics, denial, cognitive distortions, victim awareness, dangerous attitudes, fantasy, the cycle of abuse, relapse prevention, alternative coping strategies and social skills. The focus of group sessions is threefold:

1 to provide group members with information that they can use to understand and modify their thinking and behaviour;
2 to facilitate the development of insight, emotional growth and awareness that must accompany genuine change in behaviour;
3 to provide opportunities to rehearse new thinking and behaviour.

Initially the participant must identify which of his behaviours, thoughts and feelings are inappropriate, and why. Once he understands what he is required to change he must be motivated to effect change and then be offered the opportunity to rehearse his new skills and finally be rewarded for success. The overt approval of group leaders and peers must therefore be available when appropriate.

A range of cognitive, psychotherapeutic and behavioural group work exercises have proved valuable in facilitating progress. These included artwork, written exercises, drama exercises, questionnaires and discussion activities. Action techniques such as sculpting, doubling and role play have proved particularly effective in helping members to get in touch with their feelings, develop assertiveness and social skills as well as rehearsing new behaviours. Recognition that several group members are likely to have short attention spans is also important when planning sessions.

Cycle of abuse

During his time in the group, each adolescent will continually work on and improve his understanding of his individual sexual assault cycle (Ryan and Lane, 1991). The details of personal cycles are elicited through the use of a variety of techniques including 'hot seat', role play, diary keeping and artwork such as story boards. The adolescent identifies the events that trigger the cycle, the thoughts, feelings and behaviours that occurred prior to the abuse, the distorted thinking he used to excuse his behaviour, the methods used to 'groom' or prepare his victims and the consequences of the abuse for himself and others. An individual's cycle will also form the basis of his relapse-prevention programme. He will be helped to identify the 'risk' situations, thoughts and feelings and hence the circumstances which he must learn to avoid and the occasions when he might require further help. For example, one 14-year-old was able to recognise that one of his 'risk' situations was when he felt humiliated or ignored by others. He tended to withdraw to his bedroom at such times and to use sexually inappropriate fantasy to make himself feel better. By developing his assertiveness skills and improving his self-image and confidence, this individual was better able to cope with difficult social situations. His awareness of the dangers of socially withdrawing helped him to seek out someone he could talk to when he felt upset. In this manner he began to reduce the risk of his reoffending. As part of his relapse prevention programme he contracted to avoid the company of the peer group who most frequently rejected or scapegoated him.

The 'hot seat'

Some exercises are used repeatedly in the group. One example is the 'hot seat'. The exercise requires a participant to sit in front of the group and give a detailed account of a sexually abusive act he has committed. He has to include the events and feelings that occurred before and after the abuse. Other group members are expected to challenge the individual about lack of detail or inaccuracies and to confront him regarding denial, inappropriate feelings and attitudes or lack of victim empathy. During the initial stages of a group it is necessary for group leaders to facilitate and demonstrate the methods of challenge and support required during this exercise. Once a group is well established, however, the group members often perform this exercise extremely well and the group leader's main task is to intervene only on process issues, in order to maintain a balance of challenge and support. The 'hot seat' exercise provides an opportunity to monitor an individual's progress in treatment. His responses both in the hot seat and as challenger are noted and his movement on any identified treatment goals recorded.

Abusers as victims

The literature regarding sexual abusers indicates that many adolescent sexual abusers have themselves been victims of sexual abuse (Becker and Stein, 1991; Kahn and Lafond, 1988; Sefarbi, 1990) and the experience of G-MAP indicates that most adolescents who sexually abuse others perceive themselves as abused in some way. The dilemma for many professionals is whether the adolescent who has abused should be regarded primarily as a victim or an abuser. The view of those involved in the Manchester programme is that adolescents who sexually abuse must be able to accept full responsibility for their actions. Most are likely to attempt to deny, minimise or rationalise their behaviour, and in order to bring about change, professionals must avoid colluding with any of these attitudes. To place initial emphasis on an abuser's own experiences of victimisation is enhancing his 'poor me' image and giving him messages that he is not entirely responsible for his behaviour.

Those working with adolescent sexual abusers should therefore regard them as primarily in need of treatment for their abusive behaviour, although help to understand why abusive behaviour has developed is an important component of treatment. Such help should include developing recognition of the part his own abusive experiences have played, whilst understanding that since many victims of abuse do not go on to abuse others, his past cannot be an excuse for his current behaviour. For some it will be necessary to be referred for individual work on past abusive experiences to be conducted alongside the group work, although this must be carefully timed.

One of the 15-year-olds in G-MAP consistently stated that he had only abused his 9-year-old brother because his uncle had abused him. He resisted taking responsibility for his behaviour and claimed that he could not help it. By helping this young person to recognise that his uncle was fully responsible for his abusive behaviour it was eventually possible for the adolescent to accept that he himself was responsible for abusing his brother.

The treatment involved in a sexual assault specific programme is, in any event, likely to cover many issues that relate to an individual's experience of abuse. Issues of self-esteem, power relationships, vulnerability, feelings of guilt and grief are all likely to be addressed, and participants should be encouraged to share their own experiences.

Victim empathy

Dealing with issues of victim empathy can raise many previously suppressed or blocked memories and feelings relating to an abuser's own abuse. Role plays, sculpting and artwork are used to facilitate this work. An example of how these techniques can be effective is the case of Steven, a 15-year-old who had been abused himself and who was referred for sexually abusing two young female cousins. Steven initially had a low level of victim awareness. He had suppressed the feelings that he had felt as a victim and was unable to therefore recognise that his cousins suffered any negative consequences of the abuse he had perpetrated. When asked to role-play a situation where he felt vulnerable, Steven chose an occasion when he had been bullied at school. (We do not re-enact actual abuse situations in role play, because of the danger of stimulating possible abusive relationships amongst the group members.) The role play was a powerful reminder to Steven of the feelings of fear, anger and isolation and he was able to recall experiencing many of the same feelings when he was being abused. This allowed him to begin to understand how his cousins might have felt. In a later session Steven drew a picture of his victims with their arms and legs symbolically chained, their mouths zipped shut and their brains full of fog, which he labelled as fear. Methods such as these help offenders to recognise the feelings of fear, powerlessness and guilt that prevent victims from speaking out.

The process of raising awareness of the effects of abuse on victims is assisted by information drawn from extracts from victim statements, video-recordings of survivors talking, and literature. Cognitive distortions previously used by the adolescents to deny these effects are confronted and diminished, and many are made to consider for the first time the ways in which their victims suffered and the longer-term consequences of their behaviour on others.

Cognitive distortions

In addition to the techniques described above, abusers' distorted thought processes and inappropriate attitudes are dealt with using role play, question-naires, information provision and discussion. Statements that demonstrate inappropriate beliefs are challenged and explored in group sessions. The underlying constructs are confronted and alternative perspectives are provided. Questionnaires may be given as homework assignments and later used to open discussions. Role plays where the offender adopts the role of a child's (non-abusing) parent and is then presented with distorted reasons for the abuse occurring, have been found to be particularly effective. In this role the abuser will often challenge and discredit the beliefs he previously used to minimise or rationalise his behaviour.

Sex and sexuality

Adolescent sexual abusers are often confused about sex, sexual abuse, appropriate sexual relationships and male and female sexuality. Many consider sex to be dirty, or feel that they are unable to achieve satisfactory sexual relationships with peers. It is essential to deal with these issues in order to provide them with alternative, achievable, pleasurable and appro-priate alternatives to the inappropriate methods they have adopted in order to gratify their needs. Questionnaires help to identify specific issues which are then used as a basis for discussion. Sex, sexuality, gender roles and stereotypes are discussed openly, and inappropriate attitudes or beliefs are challenged and explored. Homosexuality and heterosexuality are included in discussion and care is taken not to promote heterosexuality as the only form of appropriate sexual relationships. The treatment of sexual abusers aims to reduce abusive behaviour and to promote the meeting of sexual needs via consenting relationships with peers, irrespective of orientation.

Deviant fantasy and arousal

The precise role of sexual fantasies in the aetiology of sexually abusive behaviour is yet to be established, although we appear to be on firmer ground in identifying its relevance to the maintenance of such behaviours. In therapeutic terms the challenge we face is to overcome the strong resistance most adolescents have to admitting their fantasies, particularly in a group work setting. It is often most effective to introduce an exercise in which an individual, who has previously admitted having inappropriate fantasies, for example during assessment, models an open response to other group members. The demonstration then acts to encourage other group members to provide a similar level of response. Individuals are encouraged to recognise that frequent inappropriate fantasies are a 'risk' signal which indicates that they require help and strategies for control. It is not appropriate to conduct in-depth work on sexual fantasies within the group setting, due to concern that individuals could develop and extend their own fantasies from hearing the details of others. Individual work is therefore conducted on eliciting details of sexual fantasies and providing techniques for controlling inappropriate fantasies and arousal. The central therapeutic method used in the G-MAP programme is covert sensitisation, as described by Ryan (Ryan and Lane, 1991). The difficult ethical considerations and resource implications of employing other techniques, such as the masturbation satiation as described by Becker *et al.* (1989), have meant that this is an area of work which G-MAP is still developing.

Relapse prevention

An adolescent remains in the group until it is agreed by all involved in the treatment system that the individual has achieved his identified goals. In most cases this will require an adolescent to remain in group for an average of one to two years. When an adolescent is considered to be nearing the end of group treatment he is involved in individual work and helped to draw up a relapse prevention plan. The plan is produced after consultation with the adolescent, group leaders, other group members, the key worker and others involved in his support network. The adolescent provides regular feedback to the group on his progress.

The individual's assault cycle is used to identify potential risk situations, thoughts, feelings and behaviours that the adolescent must try to avoid. Escape strategies are planned and rehearsed for future risk situations. Individuals who the adolescent can contact when 'at risk' are identified and the adolescent is invited to return to the programme at six-monthly intervals or earlier if necessary to review the plan. Those in the individual's support network, such as carers and extended family members, are involved in devising the plan and they are informed of behaviours to look out for and suggestions are made about the action to take if they are concerned. The adolescent spends several weeks establishing and rehearsing the plan before he leaves the group.

It is important that when the adolescent leaves the group he does not consider himself 'cured'. He is expected to understand that he will always remain at risk of exhibiting abusive behaviours. The prevention of reabuse will depend to a great extent on the individual's honesty with himself and others. The importance of maintaining a support network of individuals who are aware of the individual's abusive history and who are able to accept the possibility that he will reabuse is emphasised.

Progress evaluation

An individual's progress, or lack of it, is continually monitored in the group and from feedback provided by key workers and carers. The pencil and paper measures used during the formal assessment phase are also reapplied during treatment. The objective is to identify changes across a range of behavioural, cognitive, attitudinal, social and emotional factors. A paper review is completed every three months and a formal review meeting is held every six months on each participant, which involves the adolescent, his key worker, parents, carers and group leaders.

The individual's progress in each of his identified treatment areas is considered. These are likely to include:

- level of denial, ability to take full responsibility for abusive behaviour;
- capacity for victim empathy;
- ability to identify components of individual assault cycle;
- ability to identify 'risk' signals and to take avoiding action or seek appropriate help;
- openness and honesty when discussing fantasies and behaviour;
- improvement of self-esteem;
- development of assertive behaviour;
- improvement in understanding of and attitudes towards positive sexuality;
- ability to correct distorted thinking patterns;
- positive social interaction with peers;
- positive interaction with family.

Progress in these areas is noted and treatment goals are reviewed and modified as necessary. The need for individual work is examined, together with any changes or restrictions outside group that are required.

Individual work

Groupwork is the focus of treatment in this programme, but it is recognised that group treatment alone does not meet the needs of individual adolescents, their families and victims. An individual may need to concentrate on a specific area of work that is outside the group's agenda, or may need to spend longer on specific issues than the pace of the group allows. Due to time restrictions, G-MAP staff are often not able to conduct the individual work required in these cases. Often arrangements are made for the work to be undertaken by key workers or other appropriate professionals. In these circumstances close liaison with G-MAP staff is essential.

Family work

Knopp *et al.*'s survey (1992) found that 90 per cent of treatment provided to young abusers included some form of family therapy component. This makes sense, when we consider that adolescents are not operating in a vacuum. For a weekly treatment programme to be at all effective it is essential that the work is supported and maintained by others in the young person's day-to-day network. Parents and carers must play a crucial role in this task, and their inclusion and involvement in the programme is therefore important. Parents/carers need to be informed of the aims and methods of the programme and advised as to how they can best support the work that is being done there. Regular exchange of information, views and concerns is promoted via the review system and the key worker.

An adolescent's identified goals are likely to include a requirement for change in his relationships with family members and/or carers, and work that involves parents and carers may be necessary. In a number of cases families may require additional support and/or therapy to address issues which are viewed as non-conducive to the adolescent's progress – for example, where the family demonstrate denial, poor communications, inappropriate beliefs or attitudes, etc. In these cases a focused programme of family therapy is recommended and the family is referred to an appropriate resource.

Dyad work with the adolescent and family members or even his victim may be necessary during later stages of treatment. This work, however, should only be used if it is considered to be beneficial to all concerned and when all those involved agree that it is appropriate.

It is essential that those conducting treatment of adolescent sex abusers maintain strong links with other professionals who may be working with other family members and victims. This ensures that work with the abuser does not conflict with work or plans for others. It also provides for the exchange of information that might, for example, be used to confront an abuser's inappropriate beliefs and attitudes regarding his victim or family members.

CONCLUSIONS

If this chapter has had a particular constituency in mind, it has been those practitioners currently considering, planning or implementing a community-based programme for adolescent sexual abusers. Within the constraints of space we have sought to establish a framework both of the emerging knowledge base and the core components of any programme. Programmes such as G-MAP should not be considered a complete response, because of the limitations of time and resources that have been encountered. It is our view that group work programmes should, as a matter of course, be complemented by greater facilities for individual and family work than we can currently provide.

Additionally there are a number of research and practice issues which need to be addressed in working with adolescent sexual abusers, if our knowledge and effectiveness are to improve. The NCH Committee of Enquiry report (1992) effectively identifies current research needs as:

- a systematic approach to the collection of incidence data;
- evaluation of various treatment methods and techniques;
- models of causation;
- theories of normal and problematic sexuality.

Work with adolescents who sexually abuse others has only significantly emerged in the United Kingdom in recent years. We need to continue to expand our knowledge and practice base and to learn to target limited resources into methods that offer the most benefits. This will only be feasible with an approach that is research-led and which accepts the need for an in-built process of evaluation.

Many innovative developments are generated by committed individuals initiating small-scale projects. Whilst such projects are essential in identifying new areas of need or working methods, they cannot constitute a coherent service which requires a framework of resources and policy. Unless there is a shift to bring this area of work into the mainstream of practice, it appears likely that many current innovative projects will dissolve in the face of staff being given insufficient time, resources and support.

The field is on the brink of formalising and clarifying the work of the past few years. The work to date has challenged dominant ideologies, untangled a web of myths and broken the silence about sexual abuse by juveniles. As future developments refine and clarify present knowledge, the potential exists to provide a safer society by providing effective responses to sexual abuse and eventually the prevention of sexual offending.

(Ryan and Lane, 1991)

8 Parent, partner, protector
Conflicting role demands for mothers of sexually abused children

Gerrilyn Smith

Offender work is a crucial part of an overall strategy to protect children. However, it is not uncommon for those sex offenders who do undergo treatment to return to families which have had little or no work undertaken with them. This chapter describes a model recommended for use in the establishment of an appropriate protective framework by concentrating on the prevention of reabuse. It focuses on the issues involved in working with the family, particularly the non-abusing parent. As in most cases identified to date this is a female, the non-abusing parent is assumed here to be the mother. Non-abusing is not synonymous with protective, but is used to mean not having actively participated in the sexual abuse of the children. She may have failed to protect, and she may have known about the abuse. Some key issues presented should be transferable to other sexually abusive situations, for example in families where the offender is a stranger or another child of the family, and where there may be two non-abusing parents.

Whilst reference will be made to issues of race and gender, much of this chapter will be based on experience with white families where the father figure has offended against boys or girls or both. Research regarding the impact of cultural and racial differences on the manifestations, discovery and later consequences of sexual abuse for members of ethnic minority communities is rare, and generalisation across cultural and racial groups should be made with caution (Cross, 1991). Frameworks incorporating culturally sensitive means of child protection are still being developed. When considering use of the various models of assessment and treatment, therefore, workers should assess how applicable they will be across the important variables of race and gender.

SYSTEM RESPONSE

Unfortunately we still work within a child protection system which is organised around offenders. This means that resources, even in child protection agencies, are concentrated on the identification of sex offenders. Figure 8.1 provides a representation of an 'offender-organised system' and how it can move to become a 'child-centred system.' Before the sexual assault is disclosed and the offender identified, children are surrounded by a network of adults that contains both possible protectors and possible abusers. At this stage it is likely that the offender will have organised the environment, which includes the family, so that he is emotionally and physically closest to the child and any possible protectors are further away. This is the 'groomed' environment (Wolf, 1984). Any treatment programme, having identified a sex offender, should work towards empowering the possible protectors and placing them between the child and the identified abuser (stage c in Figure 8.1)

Finkelhor's four-factor model (1984) (see Chapter 1) is useful in promoting an understanding of what contributes to any sexually abusive behaviour. The model, as it is visually represented, however, appears to suggest that the largest obstacle to overcome is the child's resistance. By redrawing the diagram (Figure 8.2) it can represent a different distribution of responsibility for sexually abusive behaviour, representing the child's own resistance as the smallest impediment to abuse. Rather than Finkelhor's original representation, with smooth unbroken lines from the motivation to sexually offend through to the abusive episode itself, we need to conceptualise the offender's behaviour as a series of breaches or boundary violations. These violations represent points at which treatment services are most appropriately targeted. In a family where sexual abuse has occurred there may be an offender, a non-abusing parent and at least one target child, all of whom require some help to deal with the sexual abuse.

By using this model to develop services, an Area Child Protection Committee can identify, and assist in co-ordinating, the work of lead agencies for each of the key components of a comprehensive assessment and treatment programme. Offenders, who have both a motivation to sexually abuse and have overcome their own internal inhibitors, are dealt with primarily by probation, forensic psychiatry, psychology and prison services, and the interventions are therefore focused on Factors 1 and 2 of the Finkelhor model. Social services departments necessarily rely mainly on non-abusing mothers as external inhibitors (Factor 3 in Finkelhor's model) being more effective in preventing sexual abuse from recurring. Sadly, despite non-abusing mothers being the prime external inhibitors, the amount of training and resources allocated to this area of work is woefully inadequate and under-researched (Hooper, 1992).

Social services departments have a statutory responsibility to investigate

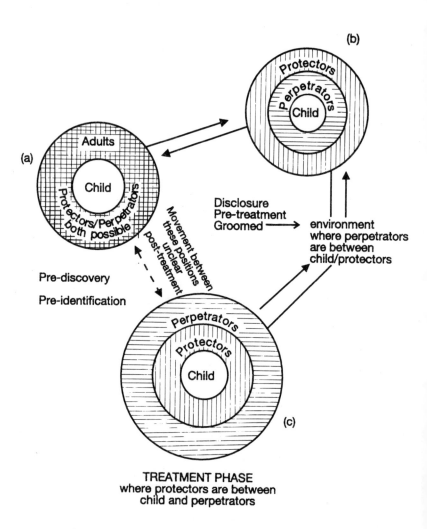

Figure 8.1 The offender-organised system: keeping it child-centred

allegations of sexual abuse which shapes much of their service provision. It is important that sufficient attempts are made to establish whether there is a non-abusing parent who might usefully be recruited to help with the investigation and who has the capacity to protect. Of equal importance, agencies need to recognise that external inhibitors may include not only mothers but also extended family members, other adults in daily contact

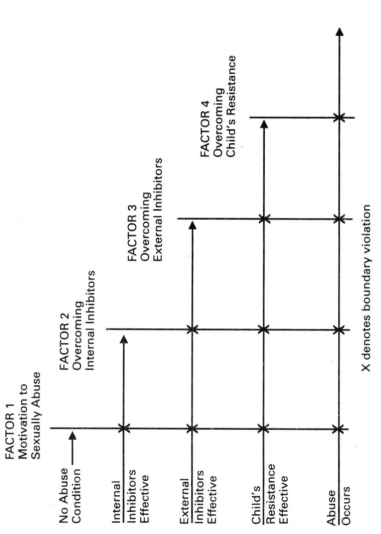

Figure 8.2 Finkelhor's four preconditions, adapted by Gerrilyn Smith

with children, such as teachers, and alternative carers of children, who may include non-custodial parents, foster carers, and residential staff. It is appropriate that social services take a lead role in developing services that strengthen the part that these people can play in inhibiting the offender's opportunity to reabuse.

In order to be effective, work will need to be multifaceted, employing a range of approaches including individual, group, and family work. The child should remain the central focus and the pace should be dictated by the child's reparative work. Unfortunately this is not the case if timescales are defined by the length of the offender's treatment, as part of a probation order or prison sentence. This may not take into consideration the time needed by the child for recovery, or the time the non-abusing parent may need in order to feel confident in both her capacity to protect and her ability to fully exercise her parenting role in other respects. A child who has been sexually assaulted will need help to recover from the experience of abuse. Ideally, this will come from the non-abusing parent, though many children will also require professional help. Additional work will need to be undertaken between the parents to consider, if appropriate, how any contact or rehabilitation between the offender and the children in the family will occur. Work is also required between mother and children together, in the absence of the offender, both because it may be some time before a decision can be reached by the mother regarding the future of the family unit, and to allow her to become re-established as an authority figure in her own family. It is most likely that the mother will need some time either on her own or with other women in a similar situation. Mothers of sexually abused children have identified particular factors that they found useful in coming to terms with the experience:

1   time to work through their feelings;
2   support that they had done the right thing by disclosing the sexual abuse;
3   being strong for their child;
4   having paid work outside the family;
5   being able to see the positive consequences from the disclosure.

(Hooper, 1992)

In some instances the mother may require both individual and groupwork and in these settings she may appear to have resolved many of the issues. It is, however, important that child protection workers see her progress translated into practice with her children. If a parent is not capable of developing or carrying out a protection plan that is developed with them, workers must reassess the level of risk to the children, which may mean considering their removal. If rehabilitation of the offender to the family is being considered, the children need to experience that both parents are behaving differently. This will require a father to acknowledge and take responsibility for his sexual offending and a mother who is able to step in and set appropriate limits if necessary. This highlights the importance of emphasising parental responsibilities in helping mothers to cope with the discovery of sexual abuse in their family.

ASSESSING A NON-ABUSING PARENT'S CAPACITY TO PROTECT

Assessing a non-abusing parent's capacity to protect is a priority for resources which, in the author's view, should take greater precedence than direct work with children. If this is not done it indirectly communicates disqualification of the most significant adult in the child's life, the non-abusing parent. The earlier discussion of Finkelhor's model serves as a useful reminder that the child's resistance to any future sexual abuse should be viewed as the smallest part of any protection package. Additionally, the child's recovery from past abuse should not be seen as the sole source of protection from future abuse.

The non-abusing parent's ability to participate openly in the assessment is likely to be improved if the assessment takes place with the alleged offender out of the family home. If this is not possible, the assessment work needs to be done with the non-abusing parent on her own, separate from the alleged offender. If the alleged offender is still in the house, there is a continuing level of risk of further episodes of abuse. If he refuses or does not allow any work with his partner or children without being present, the level of risk is higher still. It tells child protection workers there is little room for manoeuvre in this family and that the likelihood of an effective protector being empowered to act is minimal.

Someone who is suspected as an alleged offender cannot also be assessed as a potential protector. This can happen when both parents have been involved in sexually abusing their children. Workers sometimes feel that the mother, once separated from the father, poses no risk. This would need to be assessed by sex offender treatment specialists. Only in a minority of cases could a mother who was involved in sexually abusive acts with her partner be assessed as a potential protector.

The following areas are important in helping assess a non-abusing parent's capacity to protect. They will also identify a parent's strengths and weaknesses, as well as areas for change, thus providing an outline for a therapeutic programme which should follow. Although this assessment framework has been devised specifically with reference to mothers as the non-abusing parent, it could also be used with parents of children who have been abused by strangers, siblings, foster parents or residential staff.

Table 8.1 Non-abusing parent's capacity to protect

Area of assessment		Continuum of functioning				
		Optimum	Minimalising ⟷	⟷	Disbelieving ⟷	Dismal
			Movement over time			
Position regarding child's disclosure	(a) immediately (b) over time	Belief	⟷	⟷	⟷	Denying
Feelings towards child following disclosure	(a) immediately (b) over time	Empathic	⟷	Confused ⟷	⟷	Scapegoating
Role in the disclosing process		Brought concerns to attention of others	Excluded by others ⟷	⟷	Delays in bringing concerns to light ⟷	Explicitly concealed
Position regarding responsibility for abuse	(a) immediately (b) over time	Adult/ perpetrator responsible	⟷	Apportions blame ⟷	⟷	Child seen as responsible
Perceived options	(a) immediately (b) over time	Range of protective options perceived	Limited options perceived and acted on ⟷	⟷	Limited options perceived and not acted on ⟷	No options perceived. Learn to live with it

Table 8.1 Continued

	Optimum			Dismal
Cooperation with statutory rights	Alerts statutory agencies: actively cooperates	Has good reason to avoid statutory agencies, seeks alternative support	Complies with statutory agencies	Refuses to cooperate
Relationship history	Degree of independence demonstrated by periods of living alone/separate	Degree of independence not tested by separation	High degree of dependency not involving violent, abusive partners	High degree dependency involving abusive partners
Openness regarding sexual abuse in nuclear family, community and support network	Clear age-appropriate discussion with nuclear family. Appropriate involvement of extended family, support network, community	Hesitant, tentative or unclear involvement of wider network, nuclear, extended family		No discussion, keep private or promotes alternative explanations widely
Own abuse history	Previously disclosed but has worked out own resolution including self-protection	Disclosed, previously not supported, still confused, unresolved but not currently being abused		Still secret, abuse may still be going on; previous disbelieved or retracted disclosures; contact with abuser continues
Vulnerabilities such as disability	Connected to a support network (that reduces vulnerability) which is used effectively to discuss sexual abuse	Has outside support network but not able to raise concerns (re: sexual abuse)		Isolated, disconnected from an outside support network. Dependent on alleged perpetrator due to disability

Table 8.1 represents a continuum of functioning, and indicates that there may be movement over time both back towards the dismal end and forward towards the more optimal end of functioning. Notwithstanding the resource constraints outlined in Chapter 2, the Department of Health's *Protecting Children* (1989) allows approximately 12 weeks for an assessment. The author's experience is that in this amount of time it is reasonable to expect some shift towards more optimal functioning. In families where there is a high degree of suspicion, or where a clear disclosure has been made by the child, professionals should expect mothers to be functioning, at best, in the mid-range. Many offenders will have spent considerable time undermining maternal authority and creating a distance between the child and their mother. If a mother functioning initially in the mid-range has moved more to the dismal range in this period of time, this will be an indicator of the need to reassess the level of risk to the child.

The first two areas of assessment in the non-abusing parent are the priorities for change. On first contact workers may find a non-abusing parent to be minimising or possibly disbelieving of the disclosure. Professional intervention should aim to help the non-abusing parent believe the child has been or is likely to have been sexually abused. However she may still remain confused regarding her feelings towards the child and may also minimise the abuse, for example by accepting the offender's distorted account of events. A parent who believes the child from the outset is already in the optimum range of functioning. A believing adult, preferably one who lives with the child, is the first prerequisite of any protection plan. In the absence of this, it may not be safe to leave a child or children at home for the duration of the assessment.

Position regarding the child's disclosure

If the child has made a clear disclosure of sexual abuse, what is the mother's immediate response? Clearly this will be affected by the manner in which she was involved in the interviewing process. Using the child's statement can be helpful as it gives the mother the opportunity to come to terms with what the child has experienced.

The child's statement needs to be the focal point of the work for all members of the family. It needs to be viewed as more than a piece of evidence in a criminal prosecution, and should be available to treatment workers. The ACPC has an important role in facilitating the exchange of important documentation such as this. If there is no disclosure but a high index of suspicion of sexual abuse, how far is the non-abusing parent open to the possibility that sexual abuse may be the most likely explanation for the child's current behaviour problems?

What information does the mother require to move her from a disbelieving position? An offender who admits to sexually abusing his children makes it easier for a mother to believe. However, together both parents may minimise what has taken place unless workers help the mother strengthen her relationship to her child and help the child to continue to reveal what happened.

Feelings towards the child

Following disclosure of sexual abuse, workers need to assess the non-abusing parent's feelings towards the child. It is to be expected that a non-abusing parent will experience a range of feelings from sympathy to anger, although the overriding one may be confusion.

Part of a mother's confusion may come from her surprise at how the child appears to feel. Many mothers think the child should feel angry, or be more upset. They may be confused because the child demonstrates a positive attachment to the parent who has offended against them. If they believed they had a close emotional relationship with their child, they can be shocked to discover that something so significant could have escaped their attention. They will need time to understand how the child has both been taught that their feelings do not matter and has learned to keep them secret.

Role in the disclosing process

Unfortunately the mother's role in the disclosing process can be ignored, or worse, actively discouraged. At a time when, therapeutically, mother and child need to be brought closer together, professional intervention can push them further apart. It is important that those mothers who are able to respond appropriately be included in the investigative process in a manner that is ultimately most helpful for the child at a time when their belief, help and support could make all the difference to the child's long-term prognosis (Everson *et al.*, 1989). An appropriate response would include all or some of the following factors:

- the mother brought her concern to the attention of the statutory agencies;
- she is able to understand her child's need for preparation work for the medical and investigation;
- she understands why it may not be appropriate for her to sit in, but nominates an appropriate alternative protector for her child;
- she demonstrates that she can act on advice/requests from child protection workers.

Position regarding responsibility for sexual abuse

This is of less importance than her belief that sexual abuse has happened. Indeed, if she is able to discuss who is responsible for the sexual abuse there is at least an acknowledgement that it has taken place. However, blaming the child may compromise the child's position within the family if it is sustained and not modified by direct intervention that seeks to re-apportion blame in a more appropriate fashion (Elton, 1988). Clearly an admitting offender would be helpful in this matter by taking full responsibility for the behaviour. Additionally, through treatment, the offender may be able to explain to his partner the ways in which he manipulated the situation to make it appear that the child was responsible for the sexual abuse. This work will need to take place separately between the couple before a clear parental statement can be made to the children regarding adult responsibility.

Workers should expect non-abusing parents to be in the mid-range of functioning on this dimension. They may be apportioning blame not between the child and the offender, but between themselves and the offender. A clear message from the professional network needs to be given that the responsibility for the sexual abuse rests with the offender.

Perceived options

What protective options did the non-abusing parent perceive at the point she became concerned? Unfortunately the media coverage of sexual abuse investigations continues to undermine the public's confidence in the child protection services (Butler-Sloss, 1988). This has very serious consequences for non-abusing parents considering protective options in suspected sexual abuse cases. It is no surprise then that many families, and indeed whole communities – for example ethnic minority communities – would rather implement their own solutions to sexual abuse than experience the intervention of statutory agencies.

However, any attempt to resolve the problem of sexual abuse must begin with the recognition that it has happened. In order to understand the mother's response to this concern, workers need to explore her understanding of the nature of sexual abuse. Societal views that sexual abuse is about poor impulse control or that it is a transient problem are still common. If this is how the problem is understood, the solutions generated will be based on these assumptions, probably to little effect. It is not appropriate then to assess an individual as not having the capacity to protect if the solutions she was attempting to implement were entirely consistent with her understanding of the problem, even if that understanding is inadequate or inaccurate.

When assessing her capacity to protect it is also important to note that in some cases the child's mother will have sought help from outside sources but been given professional advice that allayed her fears. If there is clear evidence of professional undermining of her capacity to protect, she should not be penalised for it.

Cooperation with statutory agencies

Once a statutory agency becomes involved, to what extent does the non-abusing parent cooperate and actively participate in the protection programme? A cooperative approach is very much encouraged by the 1989 Children Act and *Working Together* (Department of Health, 1991). Workers will need to demonstrate they have made every effort to engage a non-abusing parent. By far the most difficult situation, however, is when a non-abusing parent merely complies with statutory involvement. In sexual abuse cases this can be seen when separation of the offender from the family is brought about by outside authority, rather than being a decision the woman has made herself.

This emphasises the need for workers to set clear child protection goals for the non-abusing parent, preferably observable, and to see those skills demonstrated. If the communication is satisfactory and the supporting behaviours are congruent with the verbal messages, child protection workers can accept that some degree of protection is present.

The wider cultural implications of sexual abuse may be an issue that workers from outside an ethnic minority community will find difficult to assess or even appreciate. The fears of a mother from such a community of being dealt with insensitively by a predominantly white agency, or of the response of her own community, may make it difficult for her to engage cooperatively in a protection plan. Additionally, placing her in such a central position *vis-à-vis* outside authorities may violate certain rules within her community. It is vital that professionals have access to cultural consultation when working cross-culturally.

Relationship history

In many investigations, where an offender denies committing any sexual offences, it is the mother who is given the most difficult choice by child protection agencies – to chose between her partner and her children. This is an extremely difficult choice for any woman to make, not least because of the social and economic consequences of single parenthood.

When confronted with this decision a woman can only realistically make a choice if she has experience of living separately, which would at least have given her an experience of managing on her own. However, this is not a common experience. Equally, living alone as a single woman is a very different experience from single parenthood with a child or children who may be bereft of their father and probably traumatised by his abuse of them.

A woman with a high degree of dependency on male partners, to the extent that almost 'any man will do', and a history of violent and abusive relationships, is functioning within the dismal range. She may believe her children, but often she also believes sexual abuse and violence are an inevitable way of life and consequently raises her children to learn to live with, or accommodate it (Summit, 1983).

Unfortunately an enforced separation from the offender may have only limited impact because her level of dependency would suggest that a new partner will need to be found to fill the gap. Mothers with histories of this type of relationship pattern will need more intensive work and other resources such as day centre facilities.

Communicating about the sexual abuse

It is most likely that workers will find a degree of hesitancy in the ability of non-abusing parents to talk about the sexual abuse. They will need help to decide who to appropriately tell about what has happened. This needs to be handled sensitively and in a manner that does not violate the child's privacy but alerts the child's protective network in a way that will facilitate future protection.

Mothers are often uncomfortable about telling their other children. However, to keep it secret increases the risk for these children in the event that rehabilitation of the offender is considered. They need to be aware of the problem, and empowered to tell if their father breaks agreements about his behaviour that have been made.

Any protection programme must involve a component of talking about the sexual abuse to a range of different people, including children within the family, selected extended family members and believing adults outside the family. Talking to the children should be age-appropriate and have protection as its primary focus. It is appropriate for child protection workers to discuss who needs to be told what with the child's mother. This leads to a necessary and useful discussion regarding the differences between secrecy, privacy and confidentiality. It can be helpful for the mother to know who knows what about her child. This may identify additional sources of support for her. It is important to guard against over-disclosing, or indiscriminate telling by anyone involved (i.e. children, siblings, parents or professionals).

History of sexual abuse

Research indicates a relatively high occurrence of sexual abuse in child-hood (Kelly, 1991), and that a disproportionate number of female victims have children who are themselves sexually abused. For such mothers, discovering that their own child has been abused may reactivate memories or unresolved issues from their own abuse, making it difficult for them to empathise or respond appropriately to their own child. They may also have disqualified suspicions as echoes from the past, rather than recognising them as justified suspicions about the present.

If a mother perceived herself as a protecting parent, this discovery will be particularly devastating, and she may also compare herself to her own mother, whom she may perceive as not having protected her. It will be important for workers to know how this woman's mother responded to the disclosure of sexual abuse in the previous generation.

If assessment indicates that the mother's own experience of sexual abuse requires further individual and/or group work, this needs to be provided. However, child protection agencies also need her to continue to act as a parent whilst she undertakes this work, and it is therefore important to find ways to assist her to work on childhood experiences, whilst continuing to be a capable and protecting parent. A minority of children continue to be victimised by the original perpetrator into adulthood. Such continued abuse may remind the non-abusing parent that she is not in control of her life. Additionally some of her children may have been conceived in the context of this ongoing sexual abuse. Workers should be alert to this possibility, as it is one of high risk both to the mother herself and to her children.

Other vulnerabilities

Mothers may have other vulnerabilities that the offender recognised would increase their dependence on him and facilitate the targeting and grooming process. Physical disabilities, including hearing and visual impairments, chronic physical illness, psychiatric illness, or any condition which isolates a woman from independent help, increase the possibility of exploitation and reduce her available options if she has concerns. Indeed, many sex offenders will have been admired as caring partners to these vulnerable women. They will have cultivated this dependence and may have been party to actively increasing these vulnerabilities. Professionals now recognise that children with disabilities can also be targeted by sex offenders (Kennedy, 1989). There is therefore a need to extend this work to include recognising the vulnerability of women with disabilities to targeting by sex offenders as possible partners.

Summary

All this work assumes that the non-abusing parent is making the transition to becoming a protective parent. If assessment indicates that this is not possible, then it is important that the child protection agencies put the needs of the child first. Children have strong connections to their families of origin, but they also have a right to be protected. The decision to delegate to the child responsibility for protecting him or herself should be taken only in exceptional circumstances, usually when the child is old enough to realistically take charge of his or her own protection plan and to fully understand the potential consequences of such a decision.

TREATMENT WORK WITH NON-ABUSING PARENTS

When the non-abusing parent has been assessed as having reached the minimum necessary level of protectiveness, sufficient to indicate that the children will be safe in her care, plans can then be made to undertake therapeutic work with the different levels of the familial system that have been affected by the sexual abuse. The following tasks are based on the Finkelhor model (Finkelhor, 1984) and can be categorised into the following main areas:

- providing specific knowledge regarding sexual abuse;
- developing communication skills, specifically regarding risk situations;
- developing the ability to recognise risk situations;
- reducing emotional congruence to abusive experiences;
- managing sexual behaviour;
- developing and rehearsing internal inhibitors.

Each of these tasks should then be adapted to the appropriate individual family members – children (including both the abused child and their siblings, who may not have been abused), non-abusing parent and offender. Work will need to be undertaken with each member independently, in dyads and finally, if appropriate, all together. Much of the work may be simultaneous. This is resource-intensive and requires a minimum of three workers per case – one for the abused child, one for the non-abusing parent and one for the offender. These workers should be drawn appropriately from the constituent agencies of the child protection network. In the next section, treatment work with the non-abusing parent is outlined.

Knowledge regarding sexual abuse

A non-abusing parent needs to have general information about sexual abuse. Like many members of the community, she may have misconceptions about the nature and incidence of sexual abuse. Working with a non-abusing parent and trying to understand her view about sexual abuse generally will help the professional network make more sense of her response to the disclosures made by her child.

Child protection workers should try to establish the non-abusing parent's general level of understanding about sexual abuse before moving on to look at the specific issues highlighted by this particular experience of abuse. It is also important to remember that the mother will be in shock and will require both time and support to come to terms with the abuse (Hooper, 1992).

The non-abusing parent also needs to understand how the child protection services work so that there can be a partnership between her and the agencies. (See, for example, *Through the Maze*, 1991.) Information about what will happen next is vitally important. This also includes what options are available for the family. Advice about how she may best help her child is also useful – for example: 'Your child needs to know if you believe them, whether you are angry with them.' Ideally, a parent should convey a desire to know what, if anything, has happened.

Communication skills

Whilst many professionals recognise the child's need to talk about the abuse, less commonly recognised is the same need in the non-abusing parent. She can be helped to talk about it by talking with other adults as well as her children. She may want to re-examine her listening skills. Many mothers do notice something isn't right at times with both their child and their partner. However, it is often only with hindsight that sexual abuse provides the explanation. Did the child try tell them? Did they pick up signs of the child's distress? Workers need to be sensitive to the range of possible responses a non-abusing parent might have to the communications of a child.

It is important to remember that the offender will have spent a significant amount of time preparing the environment to facilitate his offending behaviour. This includes making sure the child will keep the abuse secret. Frequently threats will have been made by the offender regarding the consequences of telling; the non-abusing parent needs to know what these may have been.

Children are often confused as to whom they should tell. Most non-abusing parents need help in this regard to protect the child from the negative consequences of people knowing too much or too little. The tendency is to keep abuse secret. The non-abusing parent will need to recognise that secrecy protects the offender and links with the coerced secrecy already established by him.

Having an opportunity to talk about the sexual abuse with professionals and other mothers is a beginning. It can be useful to go through some of the materials specifically designed to help parents talk with their children about unwanted touching. Mothers may also need to see/hear workers raise the issues with the children before they feel confident to carry on on their own. They may benefit from additional consultations or having contacts to use if they encounter difficulties at a later stage in the child's recovery process.

To perform these tasks often means a woman needs to have had time to think about these issues separately. Unfortunately, all too often mothers are not seen as individuals but are identified only by their role as mother. In a family where sexual abuse has occurred, the woman's role as partner and mother has been violated. Equally the requirements of both these roles are often in competition – to be a good partner and parent may require incompatible behaviours simultaneously.

Recognition and assessment of risk situations

It is important to remember that having identified one offender does not render children safe from other sex offenders. Parents need to know that a child once victimised is often at higher risk of future victimisation, and can therefore be helped by being introduced to primary prevention material regarding the recognition of risk. They will also need to increase the level of parental monitoring and supervision, especially if the child is exhibiting signs of increased vulnerability and distress.

Clearly, if rehabilitation of the offender to the family is not being considered then this work would focus exclusively on preventing further abuse by any others. It would be helpful to discuss the introduction of new partners into the family. How will the past episode of sexual abuse be discussed? If a woman's history of relationships indicates a lack of discrimination on her part, then it will be very important for treatment to concentrate on helping her avoid being targeted in future by any other sex offender.

If contact or rehabilitation is being considered, the offender should have undertaken specific work on his own cycle of abuse, including identifying his triggers and potential risk situations, which he will need to share with his partner before any family work is undertaken. Even where the offender has not received any treatment, the non-abusing parent may still feel able to recognise risk situations without the benefit of detailed work by the offender. Unfortunately this is unlikely to be effective, as the 'protection plan' will be distorted by the rationalisations that the offender has been using regarding his behaviour.

Only when the cycle of offending has been shared by the offender with the non-abusing parent, can work on resuming contact between the offender and the child be considered. The task for the parents will be to decide what are the priority needs of the child, and the mother should have some idea of how the child is feeling. What does the child need to hear from the offender? How will the offender convey to the child in a way that is safe and role-appropriate that he takes full responsibility for the abuse and for undermining the child's mother in her role as protector?

Emotional congruence

Emotional congruence refers to the experience or belief that abuse is an inevitable part of family life. Unfortunately some people believe this. Consequently the idea of living and parenting in the absence of any abuse (sexual or physical) may be a novel idea. Emotional congruence can be seen in both victims and offenders, clearly from opposite ends of the experience. However, they may both share a common belief about its inevitability and feel powerless to prevent or avoid it.

The issue of emotional congruence in the non-abusing parent is usually considered only with reference to a mother's own history of sexual abuse. It may be equally important to examine other aspects of emotional congruence. For example, if sexual offending behaviour is construed as a disability, many female partners may respond more sympathetically to helping their male partner live with his disability. Overly helpful behaviour on the part of a non-abusing parent in a rehabilitation programme may be an example of this. This may reflect the emotional congruence with the role of women as carers.

Women who have experiences of sexual abuse in childhood often believe that sexual abuse is inevitable and unavoidable. Consequently these women find it difficult to define a role for themselves as a protector. This has to be viewed in the context that there was little recognition regarding the impact of sexual abuse, or indeed its extent, whilst earlier generations of women grew up. It will be unlikely then that they will have received help as children to deal with the effects of their own abuse. Within the field of sexual abuse there is a long-standing tradition of mother-blaming that still manifests itself in theoretical material (Bentovim, 1988) and professional practice (Dietz and Craft, 1980). Despite knowledge about the premeditation of sex offenders, some professionals still maintain that some women choose sex offenders as partners, rather than recognising that the women are frequently targeted in the same manner as the children. Women 'choosing' partners presupposes women have a right to say 'no' to unwanted sexual advances.

Frequently sexual violence is part of domestic violence. Abel *et al.*'s (1987) work looking at a range of paraphilias in sex offenders clearly demonstrates that sexual interest in children is frequently coupled with other deviant sexual interests. Yet there is a paucity of literature on how this affects the partners of sex offenders.

Recalling Figure 8.1, where concentric circles represent the child, the non-abusing parent and the offender, there are situations where the non-abusing parent may literally have been between the children and the offender. Yet the resistance she offered was violated, often conspicuously and purposefully, in front of the children. Children can view their mothers as victims too, and may not feel anger towards them for failure to protect. Strong gender messages are being transmitted. Boys and girls are being taught how to treat women. This type of emotional congruence has clear links with society's generalised sexism. When physical and sexual violence occurs in ethnic minority families it will be further subject to racist stereotypes (Wallace, 1979). Treatment needs to address the wider issues of emotional congruence. If coercion and the abuse of authority are not to be the dominant style of family life, what will be?

Addressing issues of emotional congruence in treatment work must be part of a long-term treatment plan. How workers address emotional congruence will be directly affected by their theoretical orientation. However, workers should not expect to impact on this issue in a few sessions. It requires a detailed examination of the experiences that led to this kind of understanding of the way people and families interact, an active search for examples which challenge this view, and clear strategies for responding differently in the future.

Management of sexual behaviour

For the non-abusing parent, this is a very difficult area. On the one hand she may have a child with highly sexualised behaviour whom she is having to monitor and supervise, and on the other hand (if rehabilitation is being planned) she has a sexual partner who has violated their sexual relationship, who may be highly sexualised but not necessarily in relation to her.

To what extent does the sexual relationship of the couple dyad affect the parental dyad's capacity to protect? How, when, or if, the couple resume their sexual relationship is a pertinent issue, but the boundaries placed around their sexual relationship should be of more concern to child protection workers. In their role as parents, how will they manage their children's exploration of intimate physical relationships as they grow up? This is a task for all families. However, in a family where there has been sexual abuse it is made more difficult by the sexual boundary violation between parent and children.

In helping a non-abusing parent grapple with these issues it may be helpful to examine how these issues were dealt with within her own family of origin. In the light of the new material, what does she need to change regarding her approach as a parent to sexual development and relationships?

This may mean establishing clear vocabularies for body parts; being clear about issues relating to privacy in bedrooms and bathrooms; encouraging respect for personal space; being able to provide knowledge about sexual activities that is relevant given the child's experience; as well as giving children information about developmentally appropriate sexual behaviour.

Development and rehearsal of internal inhibitors

Non-abusing parents need to be clear about why sexual abuse against children is wrong. If they have minimised the consequences, they will need help to see the way such an act impacts not only on the target child but on the family as a whole. It should not be the responsibility of the child to describe the consequences of sexual abuse. A non-abusing parent who is moving towards being a protecting parent will be able to comment on the effects they have observed in the child of the abuse. She should be able to demonstrate her capacity to empathise with her child. Messages that this type of behaviour is wrong and unacceptable, and a clarity about why this is so, are important for all family members to hear. Children need to hear it from both parents, not just the offender. Unclear messages about inappropriate touching may lead children to believe that sexual contact *per se* is what is being castigated. The message may also have to be repeated at different developmental stages, incorporating and recognising the need to modify it in the light of an individual's own knowledge and experience.

Work on internal inhibitors is closely aligned to the work on emotional congruence. It relates directly to changing an individual's belief system regarding the acceptability/inevitability of sexual abuse, and actively involves them in generating alternative beliefs that will maximise protection, and where appropriate she will seek external support for those new beliefs. This is a long-term field of work aimed at changing beliefs that have been shaped by direct experience of sexual abuse.

CRITERIA FOR CONTACT AND/OR REUNIFICATION WITH AN IDENTIFIED SEX OFFENDER

In a family where the offender is undergoing treatment and renewed contact, or rehabilitation, is being considered, it is important that the child is showing signs of recovering from the trauma of the abuse. If the child is still symptomatic after a considerable passage of time since the disclosure of sexual abuse, workers need to consider the following:

- Is the child still being abused by the identified offender?
- Is the child being abused by an unidentified offender?
- Is the care being offered for this child within their family of origin adequately meeting the child's needs?
- Is the child still being psychologically abused by the offender?

The issue of contact between offender and family needs to be discussed in the family without the offender present. Workers will need to feel satisfied that individual members of the family are able to voice their opinions in this context. It can be useful, if there has been individual work with the target child, or the child has attended a group, to involve the worker who participated to act as an independent ally for the child to confide in. If reparative work with the child has been undertaken, then they should have knowledge about their bodies, about appropriate and inappropriate touching, and who to tell if they are confused, uncomfortable or do not like someone touching them. Clearly this is only a tiny fraction of the reparative task. (For a more detailed description of reparative work with sexually abused children, see Glaser and Frosh, 1988.) It is also important for children to understand that the abuse was not their fault and that future protection is not primarily their responsibility. It may be useful to examine their coping strategies and to help them devise other ways of behaving when they are stressed. Many children who have been sexually abused develop very challenging behaviours that bring them into contact both with the authorities and with child mental health agencies. It is important to make a connection between these behaviours and the original abuse.

Many children feel that they have either too little or too great a say in the rehabilitation process. In the former case, they experience the decision as one made by their parents, where they have little option but to agree with what is being proposed. In the latter case, they can feel that they are being asked to decide the fate of the family. It may also be tempting to say that rehabilitation of the offender back to the family should be considered/ attempted when the child is saying they are ready. However, this places too much responsibility on the child and also involves them in a decision regarding family life which is not role-appropriate. Adults should decide whether or not a partnership/family should continue.

The non-abusing parent must have made the transition to becoming a protecting parent. She must feel confident in her ability to identify situations that are risky and must feel able to intervene in interactions that she deems inappropriate. Her judgement regarding this should reflect professional concerns and assessment of risk. This also needs to be respected by the offender when he resumes contact or returns home. Consequently it is vitally important that resources are directed towards non-abusing parents and that rehabilitation work commences only when the mother has been able to assume a level of parental responsibility and authority that recognises the risks of living with a child sexual abuser. A rehabilitation programme that is led by the pace and progress of the offender's treatment can lead the other agencies to conclude that the necessary work is being done. However, if the other factors involved in the sexually abusive situation are not addressed, then child protection workers are relying completely on the offender to prevent any future sexual abuse from occurring. This is unsatisfactory as it places too much emphasis on successful treatment of the offender to ensure adequate risk reduction.

Renewed contact should be gradual and phased. It should be structured and have a purpose. Contact between the couple could begin quite soon after separation. This should be separate from the family and should not involve the children in major upheavals, i.e. the non-abusing parent should travel to an arranged meeting, rather than all the children being moved so the offender can come home. Contact between the offender and children, including the target child, should be supervised at first. This should involve a network of informed and protecting adults. Initially this may be professional child protection workers, but over time the responsibility for supervision of contact should be passed to the non-abusing parent. She should seek to recruit additional help from the extended family. High levels of supervision will be required to begin with. Certain activities should not be considered suitable, such as swimming, and the limits of all physical contact should be set and monitored. If public outings are undertaken, rules need to be established regarding supervision of the children when a protecting adult cannot be present.

It is important for possible protectors to recognise the often subtle forms of emotional pressure and abuse that can be brought to bear on children who have been victimised. Work with the child, the non-abusing parent and the offender should have identified some of these precursors to abusive episodes. They can include non-verbal behaviour such as gestures or facial expressions, verbal references to apparently benign material which is used to reinforce the special connection between the child and the offender, games and actual physical contact. Unfortunately some types of interaction must be permanently relinquished by families where sexual abuse has occurred, because they cannot revert to the benign following the previous perversion.

Any overt examples of disrespect and/or violation of conditions of access should terminate the session. If a possible protector does not intervene, they render themselves impotent and convey that impotence both to the child and the offender.

The professional network should also be clear about what progress the offender should have made prior to consideration of renewed contact or rehabilitation with his children. This should include (Morrison, 1993):

1 detailed acceptance of responsibility for the feelings, thoughts and actions which led to and sustained the abuse;
2 understanding the harm caused by his offending behaviour and the completion of a satisfactory apology to his victim and his partner;
3 some recognition of the need to change controlling and egocentric approaches to family relationships;
4 a demonstrated reduction in and control of sexual arousal to deviant stimuli;
5 improved ability to negotiate his emotional needs;
6 control of any other addictive behaviour;
7 a relapse prevention programme that he has shared with his partner;
8 a willingness to abide by the rules set by appropriate external inhibitors and monitors, who include both family members and professionals.

If both the child and the offender are away from the family of origin, priority should be given to the child returning home before the offender. However, it may be that the child does not wish to live with the offender, whereas the non-abusing parent is committed to rehabilitation. If this is the case then work should be done to identify how the young person can maintain contact with the non-abusing parent and their siblings without having to deal with the offender.

It is important that the offender returns to a family group that has been able to work together to redefine itself in his absence. The mother's parental role will need to be strengthened. She should be functioning as a parent to her children. Her authority should be recognised and respected by the children and the offender. She should not be functioning as an older sibling, as this will allow the returning offender to operate as the only adult authority in the family.

Follow-up with the children is necessary, the purpose of which would be to give the child an opportunity to express their feelings regarding the contact. Ideally the non-abusing parent should be able to monitor this, although she may feel that the children would be freer talking to an identified worker or to a member of the extended family. Direct work with the child should have progressed to the point where children would recognise situations where they should inform the non-abusing parent. For example, an offender might ask the child to keep something secret, such as giving the child chewing gum when he knows this is not allowed. Benign as this might seem, asking the child to keep something secret from their mother, and violating a known family rule set by the mother, is disrespectful of maternal authority. It also reinforces an alliance between the child and the father that previously was an unhealthy one.

In the situation where the offender is already in the family, workers are more constrained, as he is already having a great deal of unsupervised contact with the child/children. The wider network needs to be alerted for any indicators of abuse or distress (Peake, 1989a, b). However, requesting contact with the non-abusing parent and children separately from the offender will give the workers an indication of the degree to which freedom of movement is allowed to the non-abusing parent. If severely restricted, this is a poor prognostic indicator.

CONCLUSION

The goals of treatment should be:

1 Children who are more confident, have higher self-esteem, are more knowledgeable regarding the risks of sexual abuse and have identified trusted and believing adults whom they can tell.
2 Non-abusing parents who are able to protect in future because they have more knowledge regarding the risks both generally and specifically, a closer relationship to their children and access to outside support.
3 Offenders who take responsibility for the sexual abuse, are able to verbalise that to both partner and children, take responsibility for maintaining control of themselves regarding offending behaviour and better understand their appropriate role in relation to both partner and children.
4 Families with clear generational boundaries and identified roles, access to outside sources of support and an ability to communicate with each other, who are able to bring any child protection issues to the attention of a protecting extra-familial person or agency and to demonstrate the changes that have taken place, and to raise and discuss the past sexual abuse with little prompting from professionals.

Before discovery of sexual abuse the family's functioning was organised by secrecy. After disclosure, assessment and treatment the family should be organised to ensure protection from future sexual abuse. This should emphasise aspects of nurturing, respect and care that may have been present but which became perverted and distorted by the offender's deceit. A protected environment should provide all members of the family with the opportunity to grow and develop their human potential.

9   Where the professional meets the personal

Marcus Erooga

Quis custodiet ipsos custodes?' (Who will care for and protect the carers?)

(Juvenal vi: 347–8)

During the past few years many professionals have found it professionally challenging and rewarding to engage in work with sexual offenders, and it is only more recently that we have come to consider the possibility of less desirable personal effects on workers.

The impact of working with the problem of sexual abuse can be seen as paralleling the impact of sexual abuse itself. Denial, secrecy, rationalisation, avoidance, disbelief and victim-blaming are all factors that have hindered progress in defining, acknowledging and responding to the effects of the work on professionals. There is now, however, an increasing awareness of the potential effects of working with sexual abuse, but as work with offenders is less developed than that with victims, so is awareness of the possible impact.

Describing the experience in the USA, Ryan and Lane (1991) state that:

> workers have often experienced dysfunctional impacts in their own lives without understanding the nature of their reactions . . . . 'Burnout' has been accepted as inevitable and the involved systems have accepted staff turnover as if it were beyond control . . . . The acceptance of detrimental effects has been so pervasive that little has been done to confront the problem and protect workers from 'burnout', or to identify healthy management strategies.

Whilst acknowledging the greater willingness in North American culture to share personal issues, we would be well advised to note the effect on a professional community where this work is more established. As work with offenders in the UK is still in the relatively early stages of development, it is important to consider potential pitfalls and the steps needed to create a healthy working environment. It is therefore intended that this chapter will contribute to that process by considering general causes of stress in welfare work, the particular features of work with sex offenders that contribute to stress, and suggesting a framework for addressing these issues.

STRESS IN THE HELPING PROFESSIONS

Stress is part of everyday life, although in recent years the term has become more frequently used within the helping professions, with any number of meanings. Stress results from an imbalance between demands and resources (Cranwell-Ward, 1987) – when demands or pressure are experienced by an individual as exceeding their available resources. The degree of stress experienced, and its effects, are a function of the demands upon the individual and the internal and external resources they have to enable them to cope (Weiner, 1989). Thus stress will be defined here as 'An excess of demands on an individual beyond their ability to cope' (Health Education Authority, 1988).

Signs of occupational stress

Indicators of stress vary between individuals, but include demotivation, dissatisfaction, anxiety, low mood, lethargy, sleep disturbance, difficulty in concentrating, increased demands for support, and fear of making decisions. In the longer term, stress may lead to both physical and mental ill health (depression), be a cause of interpersonal and domestic relationship problems (Beckett, 1993), or 'burnout': 'the painful realisation that they no longer can help people in need, that they have nothing left in them to give' (Pines *et al.* 1981).

For Fineman (1985), burnout represents:

1 a state of emotional and physical exhaustion with a lack of concern for the job, and a low trust of others;
2 a depersonalisation of clients – a loss of caring, and cynicism toward them;
3 self-deprecation and low morale and a deep sense of failure, clearly partly a response to extreme or constant stress.

For a variety of reasons, ranging from organisational culture to personal discomfort, the experience of being under stress is often one that those in the helping professions, or their organisations, attempt to redefine or defend against. However, writers on the subject emphasise the importance of early recognition of these stress indicators in order to respond positively and effectively (Ryan and Lane,1991; Preston-Shoot and Braye, 1991).

Such responses involve identifying problems which need to be addressed before the situation worsens, both to avoid ineffective work being undertaken, and for the well-being of the worker themselves. Stress, including burnout, is avoidable, if both agencies and individuals monitor the signs of stress and act on them before the point of overload is reached.

THE NATURE OF STRESS IN WORKING WITH SEX OFFENDERS

A Health Education Authority survey, *Stress in the Public Sector* (1988), identifies three aspects of work which may contribute to stress: the nature of the work and the social context in which it takes place, organisational and management issues, and individual factors.

Nature of the work and social context

Work with sex offenders entails being exposed to powerful emotions in an intense client/worker relationship that may involve a variety of roles for the worker – helper, confessor, rule enforcer. Such work is often long-term, without easily measured successes to reinforce efforts; it involves fundamental issues about the use and abuse of power and control, authority, discipline, and emotional pain; clients are often both resistant and deceitful; it involves dealing with a high level of distortion about issues of sex and sexuality; and the fear of failure and sense of personal responsibility in workers is often considerable, in view of the consequences of further offences.

Added to this is the social context of public attitudes to sex offenders and the management of risk within which the work takes place. Work with offenders is controversial, lacking consensus from the public, media, politicians, the judiciary or indeed between professionals themselves about how it should be dealt with. In her survey of professional attitudes toward responsibility for sexual abuse and case management, Kelley (1990) found a difference in perception between members of different professions about responsibility for sexual abuse, and varying views about appropriate consequences for offenders. The professional environment therefore contains considerable ambivalence and many potential tensions.

Organisational and management issues

Workers are able to function most effectively, fulfil their tasks and feel satisfied with their own performance, when there is a clear and purposefully designed organisational structure to operate in, and where active leadership and management are provided. The absence of leadership or confusion about tasks is likely to lead to conditions which are experienced as stressful.

In her seminal study of the way in which social institutions adapt to enable their members to contain or deal with anxiety, Menzies (1970) observes:

> The needs of the members of the organisation to use it in their struggle against anxiety leads to the development of socially structured defence mechanisms, which appear as elements in the structure, culture and mode of functioning of the organisation . . . in order to avoid the experience of anxiety, guilt, doubt and uncertainty which are felt to be too deep for confrontation.

Amongst the mechanisms identified are: depersonalisation, detachment and denial of feelings, ritual task performance structured through procedures, constant counter-checking of decisions, and avoiding change and clinging to the familiar, even when it has ceased to be appropriate.

Because of the distortions involved, these social defence mechanisms do not enable reality to be confronted and deprive staff of the necessary rewards and reassurances for their work. This then leads to poor decision making, a decrease in self-confidence and trust, and an erosion of discretion and guilt about responding in this manner. The social defence systems themselves thus become a source of secondary anxiety, or stress.

The development of work with sex offenders has been characterised by practitioner-led initiatives. Some, if not many managers have been left feeling unsure of their own knowledge base, uncertain about a potentially controversial area of work and as a consequence ambivalent, unsure or uncommitted when asked for support. Such absences of leadership and support will leave practitioners' anxieties uncontained and vulnerable to the dysfunctional coping responses identified by Menzies. The danger is that in response it may be easier to deny the discomfort, confusion and conflict than to begin to address the personal issues which work with these clients raises.

In addition, when workers develop a new initiative without clear management mandate, they can also take disproportionate responsibility for its success or failure. Organisational problems are then all too easily defined as personal failings, and initiatives ultimately discontinued, regarded as unrealistic experiments. As a result, practitioners and managers become caught up in vicious circles where cause and effect become confused and responses to problems become ineffective (Preston-Shoot and Braye, 1991).

However, if an interactional model (Morrison, 1991) is used to take account of the range of factors at work, the total context in which the work is being undertaken is clearer, and a more realistic view emerges. Difficulties and successes can then be viewed as the result of the interplay

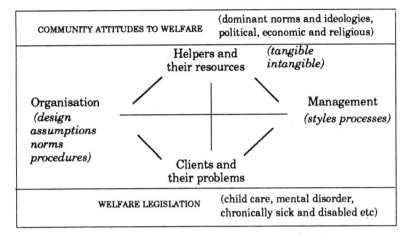

Figure 9.1 Factors contributing to dysfunctional stress among helpers

Source: Morrison, T. (1991) 'The Emotional Effects of Child Protection Work on the Worker', *Practice* 4(4): 254.

of societal, legal, interagency, agency, management, colleague, client and personal issues and it becomes more likely that a more accurate analysis of problems and solutions can be formulated. Of course, excessive emphasis on any one factor, or conversely overlooking the significance of any factor, will result in an unbalanced analysis of the problem and therefore ineffective responses. This is of particular importance, as an effective strategy of change requires responses at every level of an organisation, based on an assessment of areas where stress occurs (Preston-Shoot and Braye, 1991).

Transference and countertransference

The 'helping professions' work with a range of demanding and painful issues – illness, separation, loss, and a range of forms of abuse. In common with the other areas of work, dealing with sex offenders brings its own particular sources of challenge and stress. In addition to the specific issues outlined below, however, practitioners also need to maintain an awareness of the phenomena of transference and countertransference, as well as the functioning of their own defences.

Transference is the process by which the client transfers feelings applicable to a previous relationship into the present one between the offender and the worker, whilst countertransference can be defined as the feelings which arise in practitioners towards their clients, either in response to the transference, or as a result of the (usually unresolved) personal issues which the practitioner brings to the relationship. As one possible effect of transference or countertransference may be increased stress, it will be important that the cause of this form of stress should not be confused with those discussed below. Good supervision is vital in identifying and addressing issues of transference and countertransference.

Defence mechanisms

Defences are those mechanisms by which people alter information which is at variance with, or which threaten, their perception of themselves. In working with unpleasant or distressing material, practitioners will develop self-protective defence mechanisms. Common individual responses in child protection include professional distancing – 'It's not appropriate for me to get involved', projection – 'I'm not angry, but he's so aggressive', dissociation from responsibility or authority – 'I don't want to do this, but . . . ' and denial – 'I'm sure he wouldn't do that'.

However, as Ryan and Lane (1991) observe:

> It is initially adaptive to, and healthy to protect oneself from being overwhelmed by the experience [of being exposed to the detail of sexual offending]. It must be remembered however that coping does not equal resolution, and overgeneralisation of defence mechanisms becomes maladaptive over time.

Unfortunately, in most professions there is an absence of any culture of attending to these issues. Indeed, in many organisations a premium is placed on ability to endure difficult conditions and routinely deal with frightening or emotionally exhausting situations by exhibiting external calmness.

As well as recognising the nature of defences, therefore, there is a need to strive for sufficient self-awareness of personal and professional behaviour to identify when this is happening and take such action as is possible to maintain emotional well-being.

Individual factors in work with sex offenders

Sex and sexuality

Sex, and sexuality, are governed by ideas and beliefs as well as biological drives. By working in this area we are not only exposed to the internal worlds of sex offenders, but are likely to experience some effect on our own internal world. This effect can be partly explained by the view that

'Sexuality involves the ways in which a person defines her or himself, the definitions one makes of others, and the meanings we give to our relationships' (Petras, 1973). The ensuing re-evaluation of our ideas and beliefs is not necessarily a negative experience, but we should be aware of the possibility of this process when we commence the work. We should not expect that we can be repeatedly exposed to accounts of abusive sexuality and not experience some effect on our own sexuality.

Workers who themselves have sexual problems may become more aware of them. Workers who have themselves been victimised may have that awareness restimulated. Responses to offenders' issues may intrude on workers' sexual lives. Many report becoming disinterested in sex for a time; conversely, some report a level of arousal to aspects of the material they are working with. Workers who are also parents may become over-protective, or preoccupied by the need to keep their own children safe. Many report experiencing difficulty in working with offenders whose victims have been of a similar age to their own children, or of the same name.

Identification and fear of contamination

There is an emerging realisation that sexual offending is not confined to a deviant few, nor are offenders from particular social classes. Working with this client group, one of the most striking features is the absence of easily recognisable characteristics – there is nothing to which we can point and say, 'They're all different from me, or my partner, or my colleagues because . . . '. There is no easy mechanism by which we can distance ourselves, or those we love, from sex offenders.

This desire for differentiation from offenders is not restricted to individual workers. At a societal level, Pithers (1990) observes that

Sexual aggression has often been considered an impulsive act . . . Our safety seems less precarious if we believe sexual abuse is performed by individuals who have taken momentary leave of their faculties. Such a premise also enables us to evade recognition that many men who do not aggress sexually have momentary impulses to do so.

This is an uncomfortable reality to live with.

The proximity and intimacy of the work may also lead to a fear of contamination for practitioners concerning the 'discovery' or development of aspects of themselves similar to some of the unacceptable characteristics or behaviours of offenders. Indeed it is likely that there will be aspects of sexual offenders, as with other client groups, which are similar to workers. They will behave in ways we recognise, have some attitudes we may have once also held or have some sympathy with now. It can be disturbing if we discover that there are aspects of our sexuality which resemble that of offenders. Our fantasies and sexual behaviour, even if they involve consenting adults, may be similar to those described by offenders. The less acceptable or comfortable aspects of our sexuality may include aspects of coerciveness or exploitation which we prefer not to acknowledge.

At a social level, the response of family, friends, peers or managers may range from 'Well, I suppose somebody has to . . . ' to 'What do you get out of it?', leaving workers feeling that they are also in some way reviled, or an object of suspicion, a further form of contamination.

Exposure to dominating and controlling behaviours

Exposure to such behaviours is pervasive because of the way in which offenders use control and manipulation to manage their world (Lane, 1986). Working with sex offenders gives the practitioner direct experience of the ways in which offenders may inappropriately try to exercise control and to manipulate power in relationships. At times it may be difficult to continue to maintain a legitimate use of therapeutic and statutory authority without becoming persecutory (Sheath, 1990). Offenders' behaviour may also evoke particular responses in male and female workers, including feelings of being discounted, ineffectual, angry, helpless, powerful, or powerless. Workers therefore face stresses at two levels: the uncomfortable feelings themselves and the discomfort caused by the conflict of being a 'helping' professional and having such feelings.

Values, beliefs and principles

> Decisions on how you treat each family member depend crucially on how you theorise about them . . . Are we looking at a family pathology, a Freudian spider's web or a legacy of patriarchy? Not the smallest step in dealing with incest is free of theory.
>
> (Nelson, 1982)

Professional values do not exist independently of wider social forces and interests. As well as a need to be clear about the causes of, and offenders' responsibility for, sexual abuse, it is also important for workers to be aware of these wider influences and their own values and beliefs about sexuality, which will influence not only their practice, but also the personal impact of the work.

By developing such an awareness, it is possible to increase the ability to make sense of, and deal effectively with, the contradictory expectations, feelings and experiences workers may be subject to from 'society', their agency, their clients, partners, friends and themselves in working with sex offenders.

Gender issues

Probably the most striking feature of our current knowledge about sexual abuse is that abusers are predominantly men, who in a patriarchal society have considerable power because of their gender. Their victims are women and children who are vulnerable and less powerful than themselves in a number of ways. For workers this may raise strong feelings, some of which will depend on the gender of the worker.

Clients may make appeals to gender: 'You're a man, you understand', or behave differently with male and female workers; female workers may feel sexually threatened by a particular client in a way with which male colleagues find it difficult to identify – all of which are potentially divisive matters if not discussed and dealt with by the staff team.

> Following a group session Alice reported to her co-worker (one male and one female) that she felt 'threatened' by the way in which Gerald, one of the offenders in the group, addressed the majority of his comments to her. She found it difficult to define the nature of her discomfort, but experienced it as disempowering and thought it was his way of exercising control. Other staff had noticed the focus on Alice, but had not considered its significance. The male workers found it difficult to empathise with her experience, but trusted her perception and at the next meeting this behaviour was addressed. Gerald acknowledged that Alice reminded him of his ex-wife, to whom he had been physically violent, and that he was having sexual fantasies about her. These issues were then addressed in group sessions and individual work.

Female workers may feel covertly victimised during the process of working with offenders, or may feel a generalised anger with men for their abusive behaviour and abuse of power, or feel unable to trust any man, in view of the apparent 'normality' of many offenders. Male workers may also feel covertly victimised, have feelings of identification with offenders because of gender, experience 'gender guilt', feel blamed for their own maleness, or experience other issues related to the use of power in their own lives (Lane, 1986).

Equally important in a co-work relationship will be the ability to discuss sexual and gender-related issues openly, in order to avoid any replication of imbalanced power relationships in the co-workers' relationships. Whilst this is important in all co-work, it becomes particularly crucial when working with a client group whose own view of male/female relationships is highly distorted.

Similarly, issues of race or ethnicity may have a significant impact on workers' experience. Myths or stereotypes about different races or cultures may lead to conflict or misunderstanding, and the possibility of this needs to be acknowledged and explored at an early stage.

All of the issues outlined above can be anticipated to affect individuals and teams; it is their denial or neglect, rather than their existence, which is likely to be problematic. A structured process of debriefing and recording at the conclusion of each period of client contact, be that an interview or a group session, will be important tools in acknowledging and processing issues.

PREPARING FOR WORK WITH SEX OFFENDERS

The report of the Cleveland Inquiry (Butler-Sloss, 1988) recommended that workers should make a choice about whether or not to work with sexual abuse. Although the inquiry did not consider work with sexual offenders *per se*, the same point certainly applies. For those moving into this area, or for whom it will form some part of their work, it is important at the outset to have some awareness of what is being taken on and to consciously prepare for the work. Inevitably, not all of the potential difficulties will be clear at the outset, nor can we know how we or others will react, but time spent in considering potential issues is likely to reduce stress and uncertainty later.

The discussion which follows is primarily focused on the preparation required for workers to make a decision to specialise, or work to a significant extent, with sex offenders. It is important to acknowledge, however, that many workers involved with sexual offenders do not choose to do so, but undertake the work of necessity. It is hoped that the discussion will also have relevance for those able to exercise less choice about their involvement, but who nonetheless need to prepare for the work.

Building blocks to staff care

A useful structure within which individuals can think about the different areas which will require attention is to consider them under four headings: personal, professional, agency and co-work issues. Workers will not have equal control of issues in all of these areas. It is important, therefore, for individuals to be clear about the level of control that they do have over their potential involvement, to decide what are the essential minimum requirements for them to choose to undertake this work, possibly to resist pressure to become involved if such requirements cannot be achieved and finally to consider what they can do if involvement cannot be avoided. This section is therefore presented as a number of building blocks for staff care (see Figure 9.2), underlining the fact that the stability and sustainability of the work depend on the quality of the preparation undertaken.

Personal issues

1 **Motivation** The experience of working with sex offenders is one which many practitioners find energising and satisfying, as well as personally challenging. However, to maximise effectiveness and reduce potentially negative impacts, it is important to understand one's own motivation to work with this client group. This may be assisted by preparing a list of the reasons for wanting, or being willing, to do this work and what it is hoped to derive from the experience. This list may also be helpful in deciding how to respond when managers, colleagues, friends or offenders ask: 'Why you do this work?'

When generating the list, it will be important to consider the possibility that motivation may be based on a desire for retaliation for previous experience of abuse, or a desire to punish sexual offenders – motives which are likely to lead to rigid practice and ultimately prove dysfunctional for both for workers and offenders.

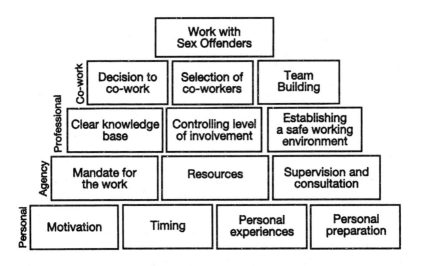

Figure 9.2 Preparation building blocks

2　**Timing**　Even for those who actively chose this work, there may be particular periods or life events when work with sex offenders becomes more problematic or difficult – for example, during pregnancy, or relationship problems.

3　**Personal experiences**　The work may evoke experiences from the past, especially for those who have been sexually or otherwise abused. Planning for ways to deal with that and considering what help – in terms of supervision or support – will be available, may prove important.

4　**Personal preparation**　All workers should try to anticipate some of the ways in which the work may impact, and whether to talk to others who may also be affected. Spouses or domestic partners may find it helpful to be told about possible responses and reassured that, for example, a temporary disinterest in, or aversion to, sexual activity is likely to be about the work, not a more fundamental relationship problem. It may be helpful to share any anxiety about not knowing what effects the work may have, and make a commitment to share important issues. The exact nature of this preparation will depend on individual relationships and situations, but some preparation in personal relationships may offer an additional source of support.

Agency issues

1　**Mandate for the work**　A key factor is having a mandate for the work at a senior level from the agencies involved. Without this, there is a danger that ignorance, misunderstanding or suspicion may lead to damaging or prejudicial managerial responses or indeed to treatment programmes being prematurely terminated and for workers feeling overly responsible (Morrison, 1992).

2　**Resources**　Workers therefore need to know what support in terms of time and resources they will be allowed, determining whether that is likely to be sufficient, and if not, attempting to negotiate for further resources. Many workers 'solve' resource problems by effectively undertaking this work in their own time, often based on agency permission to do the work as long as everything else still gets done. This should be avoided, as in the long-term it adds significantly to workers' stress and is ultimately unmanageable.

3　**Supervision and consultancy**　Within social work, supervision remains the fundamental method by which agency oversight of practice is exercised, although the need for such oversight and support is equally applicable to practitioners from other disciplines. Whilst many workers' experience of supervision is mixed, ranging from the enabling and empowering to the undermining and immobilising, good supervision is a vital contribution to workers' practice and personal well-being. Thus the Probation Service thematic inspection reports: ' . . . [in] cases where the quality of supervision was judged to be poor, staff were colluding with offenders in avoiding issues and more effective staff supervision would have improved that position' (Home Office, 1991).

However, it may be that for a variety of reasons the line manager is not the person most suitable or best qualified to provide this, and consideration may need to be given to an agreement for this to be provided by another manager, colleague or external consultant. The thematic inspection observed that 'some supervisors were not sufficiently aware that confronting sexual offending requires staff to examine their personal attitudes and behaviour – and indeed their relationships – in a way that does not apply when working with other types of offender' (ibid.). This process is unlikely to occur in a relationship which does not acknowledge the importance and effect of issues affecting power and difference, such as gender and race, within supervision.

Particular issues for women workers in supervision are the development of strength and self-esteem; empowerment to work appropriately and effectively; the ability to say 'no' and set boundaries around particular activities, or when they want to suspend or terminate their involvement; and developing strategies to reduce the personal impact of undertaking work with this client group (Cowburn and Wilson, 1992). For male workers the issues include concerns about unwitting collusion, negative feelings about male sexuality, and consideration of appropriate use of power during work with offenders.

Practitioners therefore need access to a supervisor or consultant (of the same gender if they wish) who has a knowledge of work with sex offenders, with whom there is a relationship of trust and who has knowledge of the area of work and its potential impact.

Professional issues

1 **Clear knowledge base** It will be important to develop a clear theoretical and knowledge base about the nature of sexual abuse and sexual offending, as well as about different models of treatment. This is a client group whose level of distortion about these issues is usually deep-rooted and difficult to change. Faced with this, professionals may come to doubt, albeit momentarily, what they believe themselves. Clarity and confidence in a clear theoretical base about sexual offending will help to reduce the likelihood of this happening and will also be important when working with denial. Training

therefore has a key role to play in acquiring and testing out theoretical knowledge and skills. Training courses should provide opportunities both to begin exploring these issues and meet other workers, as well as providing new knowledge and skills. Cognitive preparation and theoretical clarity is as important for empowerment as emotional preparation.

2 **Controlling level of involvement**   It may be that having expressed an interest in this area of work, practitioners unintentionally come to be regarded as the local expert on sex offenders, and come under pressure to take on all work with this client group, or to take on other consultation or specialist work. It will be necessary to make efforts, in consultation with managers, to control the level of involvement, to ensure that boundaries are maintained and to ensure that workers are not operating beyond their levels of confidence and competence.

3 **Establishing a safe working environment**   There may be particular requirements to achieve a sense of personal 'safety'. These may be physical requirements – for example, knowing that there will be appropriate facilities available – or professional support such as adequate supervision or consultancy, or the approval or support of colleagues about the work. If these are determined at this stage, they will assist when negotiating within the agency about how the work is to be undertaken.

Co-work

1 **Decision to co-work**   Co-working is an important way to reduce isolation, secrecy and stress. Kerr (1991) found that Probation Officers experienced 'comfort and reassurance' from co-working, as well as it having benefits therapeutically. However, in order for co-working to be successful, attention will need to be paid to the selection and preparation of co-workers. This is easily overlooked when two or more people express an interest in working together, in that it is not always those who like each other who make good co-workers.

2 **Selection of co-workers**

> In the world of child protection we talk about the concept of 'working together' with loose abandon, rarely unpicking some of the real difficulties involved. Somehow we assume that because we are all in the 'helping' professions, we will be 'helpful' to each other and that we are all naturally team players.
>
> (Morrison, 1990)

In order for co-work to be effective there needs first to be a process of selection based on a proper understanding of what the co-work is intended to achieve, rather than other factors such as geographic proximity or mutual availability. Thus, following an initial expression of interest it will be important to discuss aims, hopes and working styles, before a co-work pairing or team is established.

3 **Team building** The next stage is to begin to understand some of each others' values, feelings, fears, skills and behaviour. Difficult issues between workers, and between workers and offenders, will arise, and there is often a natural reticence about discussing such problems through fear or lack of awareness. Such processes need to be dealt with openly, as they are likely to become more powerful and destructive the less explicit they become. Thus, on the whole it is easier for co-workers to focus simply on the progress of cases than on the developments and strains of a co-work relationship. Conversely, it is possible to over-focus on the interpersonal issues between workers and so fail to adequately consider the clients. A balance must be found to ensure that both are dealt with.

Co-work 'teams' therefore need to prepare themselves to work together, both in terms of clinical and co-work issues. Good preparation will be the basis of effective teamwork, which in turn enables workers to perform more skilfully and confidently with their clients and to have confidence in their decisions (Erooga, 1983).

For some practitioners, 'team building' will be a familiar idea, whilst for others it will be less familiar. Essentially it is a structured process by which potential co-workers can consider their 'fit' to work together and begin to prepare for the task. As well as facilitating co-work, it offers the opportunity to explore the possibility that co-working will not be advisable before embarking on practice together. The team preparation process below is intended to offer a simple structure which can be adapted to suit the needs and preferences of those involved.

A six-stage preparation process is outlined here, based on the assumption that the issues outlined in the 'building blocks' above have been addressed at an individual level by workers. The stages may not be exhaustive, and priorities will depend on agency setting, previous history of working together, and the nature of the work to be undertaken. Some of the issues can be dealt with by the workers involved alone, whilst others will benefit from the use of an external consultant, acting as facilitator to explore the issues and offer feedback. Stages 4 and 5 are priorities for the use of a consultant. The six stages are presented as a checklist to enable their use by potential co-workers.

The six stages of preparation

1 Orientation.
2 Defining the task.
3 Contracting and agreement between workers and 'facilitator'.
4 Trust-building.
5 Problem solving.
6 Viability and maintenance.

Areas to cover

1 **Team orientation**
   — What is the course of events that have led us to be coming together to undertake this work?
   — What agency expectations and constraints are we subject to?
   — Who is accountable for this work? How is this accountability exercised?
   — Do we all have the same responsibility for this project?
   — Do we know what each other's job is? Are we of different status?
   — What effect will any differences of status have on the team?
2 **Defining the task – what are we doing?**
   — What is this piece of work? (Don't assume a common understanding of the task)
   — Why do we want to/ are we willing to do this work?
   — What are the focus and goals of the work?
   — How will they be achieved?
   — Do we all want to co-work?
   — If so, why? If not, do we have a choice about not doing so. Can we resolve this? How does this affect viability as co-workers?
3 **Contracting and agreement between workers and 'facilitator'**
   — What do the workers want from these preparation meetings?
   — What fears and fantasies do they have about the team preparation process?
   — What do the workers want and not want from a facilitator?
   — Is everyone clear about how the facilitator will be accountable to the agencies involved?
4 **Workers sharing information/building trust**
   — What values, attitudes and theoretical models do we each bring?
   — What else do you need to know about your colleague(s) to work effectively together with sex offenders? (List five things).
   — What do you need to let your colleague(s) know about you to work together?

— Have you addressed issues of difference in gender and race between you? What effect might those differences have on your work? What do you and your colleague(s) need to talk about in relation to those issues?
— What do you feel most confident about contributing to this piece of work in terms of skills, experience, etc.?
— What do you feel least confident about? What are the limits of your skills, experience, etc.?

5 Team contracting and problem solving

— How might you get into difficulties/ stuck during the work? How would your co-worker/s know?
— What help would you want from your co-worker/s?
— What would your co-worker/s want from you?
— What if you make mistakes? What permission do you need from others to make mistakes?
— What will be most difficult for you if your co-worker/s make mistakes? What permissions can you give?
— How do you think you might behave in this team (based on how you've been in other groups)? Is there anything you'd want to do differently? Do you want any help with that from your co-worker/s?
— In what ways, either consciously or unconsciously, might you undermine teamwork?

6 Viability and maintenance

— How will we know if this is a viable team to proceed with this piece of work?
— What will we do if this is not a viable team to proceed with this piece of work?
— Is this a viable team to proceed with this piece of work?
— Do we need further team preparation:
  (i)   Before deciding on viability?
  (ii) Having agreed on viability but before starting the work?
  (iii) Once the work has started?
— What will the team need to maintain healthy functioning over the period of the work (e.g. consultation; training)?

CONCLUSION

Given the potential personal impact of working with sexual offenders, it is important to consider our attitudes to self-care and to caring for colleagues, to pay attention to personal needs and to make efforts to ensure they are met appropriately and sustained over time. Most workers already have at least a notion, if not clear ideas, about how they should care for themselves and for colleagues. Too often, however, under pressure it becomes easy to stop noticing that those things are not being done. What were originally small concessions can become major compromises.

Those who are able to maintain professional and personal well-being in this work will have a healthy belief that, whilst at times it may be personally difficult, we all have a right to be emotionally well in the work we do and that we are more important than our work. At a very personal level it is also important to celebrate those aspects of our own sexuality which are non-abusive, non-coercive and non-exploitative.

Finally, as members of the 'helping' professions, we are notorious for being hard on ourselves about what we have not done perfectly. Ultimately emotional health will involve forgiving ourselves for not doing some things as well as we could and celebrating all those things that we have done as well as we can do them.

Conclusion

> The relative youth of many of the programmes and the recent high profile of sex offender treatment imply that much of this activity could stop as rapidly as it began.
>
> (Barker, 1991)

If, in twenty years time, we should review the natural history of work with sex offenders in the UK, will our current achievements and enthusiasm prove to have been merely another passing fad, kindled by a brief surge of therapeutic optimism? Will work with sex offenders remain a special interest area for a few dedicated practitioners? Indeed, some are wondering that now. Perhaps we might then look back and consider whether we laid the foundations deeply or strongly enough to sustain and develop the field?

Although we cannot know now whether the foundations will prove sufficient, this book has sought to reflect something of the achievements so far. These include:

- a multi-factorial model of aetiology which recognises the interplay of societal, environmental and interpersonal factors contributing to sexually abusive behaviour;
- the location of the work within a multi-disciplinary child protection framework with the clear overall objective of protecting children;
- the growing recognition by central government and senior managers of their roles in co-ordinating a strategic response;
- the application of research to theoretical models of intervention;
- an eclectic approach to treatment and a commitment to evaluate outcomes;
- the establishment of a national organisation, NOTA;
- the development of practice standards and the acknowledgement that for some staff this will not be an appropriate area of practice;
- the application of knowledge about sexual offenders in strengthening

the overall effort to combat sexism at personal, professional and societal levels.

We are also facing a crucial test as to whether the hard work to date in getting this work onto the professional agenda will lead to its integration within the mainstream of agency and interagency objectives, planning and provision in the face of competing priorities. Once practitioners stop undertaking this work in their own time, how much treatment will agencies be prepared to pay for?

There is, however, an even stiffer test to come: that of societal understanding, confidence and tolerance of this work. There are few votes in work with sex offenders. To date, not enough has been done to inform the public about the need to work with sex offenders. The history of British child abuse public inquiries has not been a positive one. Whilst they have undoubtedly led to major changes in both practice and legislation, there is little doubt that the process has also depressed public and professional confidence in child protection services.

In 1988 the Canadian government established a board of investigation following the sexual assault and murder of a woman by an offender who was in breach of the conditions of a temporary release from a community residential facility. This recommended that

> The Government of Canada initiate a comprehensive evaluation of the effectiveness of all present sexual offender treatment programs. If such an evaluation indicates that there are no effective treatment programs at present, further consideration should be given to ending ineffective programs and concentrating funds and human resources in those areas where such promise is shown.
>
> (Working Group, 1988)

The review concluded: 'whilst no approach can offer total success, various approaches have shown some success . . . [we estimate] treatment can be effective in reducing sexual recidivism from about 25 per cent to 10–15 per cent' (ibid.). Indeed, Marshall *et al.* (1990) comment that 'Since most recidivists offend against more than one victim, success with just 1 offender for every 50 treated can be counted as socially valuable'.

However, the Canadian review also noted the dangers of treating offenders in inappropriate programmes, due to the false perception that can be generated in the public that an offender presents a decreased risk solely by virtue of having attended a programme. It is instructive to note the similarities between many of their organisational and therapeutic difficulties and those facing British practice.

In the UK context, given the lack of public acceptance of the need to work with sex offenders, and society's natural wish to punish and distance itself from them, one wonders about the consequences of a public inquiry in circumstances similar to those in Canada. Would the public be willing to support resources being directed to such a traditionally reviled group? How far would it be accepted that treating sex offenders is a risk business? What will happen if there is a public conflict between moral and therapeutic responses? How well would the professional community be able to withstand the harsh scrutiny of such an inquiry?

We should not need to wait for a crisis of external confidence to take the next steps towards strengthening and integrating this work within both public understanding and organisational thinking and planning. It is these steps that are amongst the key challenges of the next few years. They can be considered at three levels: public, professional and personal.

At a public level, efforts must be made to inform society about the nature and pervasiveness of sexually abusive behaviour and the need to work with sex offenders. Society's wish to distance itself from such behaviour is entirely understandable, based as it is in anger, fear and helplessness. Educating the public, difficult though this will be, is vital if professionals are not unwittingly to establish a climate of unhealthy secrecy about this work. Public and politicians need to have clear and realistic expectations about what can and cannot be achieved in working with sex offenders. There are, and will continue to be, risks in doing such work, which society must either accept, or choose to incarcerate all sex offenders for life. We must also work to convince the public that our approach is both disciplined and rooted in an overriding concern for the safety of all potential victims. It must be clear that treatment is not an alternative to offenders facing public accountability for their actions. A more complex task is primary prevention – educating and engaging society about the need to change underlying attitudes and structures that support offending behaviour into which children are socialised.

At a professional level the goal is the integration of offender management within agency and interagency philosophies, structures and provision as well as within an overall response to child sexual abuse. In this context it is also vital that the management of other types of sex offenders is considered. Of immediate importance in achieving this are interdepartmental government co-ordination, the establishment of standards and guidelines, a coherent training and development framework for practitioners, prioritised service plans and outcome research.

The resource-intensive nature of offender work will continue to be a problem for agencies, and it is highly unlikely that all offenders will receive a comprehensive service. However, the development of skills in working with sex offenders will be of enormous benefit across a wide range of client groups and it is therefore hoped that senior managers will regard this work as a long-term investment in the development of a more skilled workforce.

Finally, at a personal level there are three themes which we should keep before us in this demanding and intrusive work. First, we need to be clear about our beliefs concerning the nature and causes of sexual offending against children. Second, we need to be honest with ourselves and those with whom we work about why we do this work. Finally, above all, we should never forget the enduring damage that sexual offending causes and that our overriding goal is that children should grow and develop free from the experience, or the fear, of sexual abuse.

Appendix: Appeal Court guidelines on sentencing in cases of incest

The Appeal Court guidelines laid down by Lord Chief Justice Lane were reported in *All England Law Reports* (1989) 3. They followed a referral by the Attorney General of a case where he felt the sentence, amounting to three years' imprisonment, for a man convicted of three counts of incest and one of indecent assault was too lenient. The Appeal Court increased the sentence to six years in respect of the two incest counts concerning the child, who was under 13 years of age.

The guidelines are as follows (Yates, 1990):

Where the girl is over 16

Generally speaking, a range from three years' imprisonment down to a nominal penalty will be appropriate, depending upon whether on the one hand, force was used and upon the degree of harm; and on the other, the desirability of keeping the family disruption to a minimum. The older the girl, the greater the possibility that she may have been a willing or even the instigating party to the liaison. This is a factor which will be reflected in the sentence – in other words, the lower the degree of corruption, the lower the penalty.

Where the girl is from 13 to 16

Here a sentence of between three and five years seems to be appropriate. Much the same principles will apply as in the above, though the likelihood of corruption by the man decreases in proportion to the age of the girl.

Where the girl is under 13

It is here that the widest range of sentences is likely to be found. If the girl has taken on the wife's role, is not far short of her thirteenth birthday and there are no particularly adverse or favourable features on a not guilty plea, a term of about six years would seem appropriate. The younger the child when the father's sexual advances began, the more likely it will be that the girl's will was overborne and, accordingly the more serious the crime and the longer the sentence.

Aggravating and mitigating factors

Aggravating factors include:

1   if there is evidence that the girl has suffered from the incest;
2   if the incest has continued at frequent intervals over a long time;
3   if the girl has been threatened or treated violently by, or was terrified by the father;
4   if the incest has been accompanied by perversions abhorrent to the girl;
5   if the girl has become pregnant by reason of the father failing to take contraceptive measures;
6   if the defendant has committed offences against more than one girl.

Mitigating factors include:

1   a plea of guilt;
2   if the father had genuine affection for the girl;
3   if the girl has had previous sexual experience;
4   where a shorter penalty is for the benefit of the victim or the family.

Bibliography

Abel, G. (1987) 'Surveillance groups', paper presented at the annual meeting of the Association for the Behavioral Treatment of Sexual Abusers, May, Newport, OR.

Abel, G. and Becker, J. (1984) 'Abel and Becker Cognitions Scale', in Abel, G., Becker, J., Cunningham-Rathner, J., Mittelman, M., Rouleau, J., Kaplan, M. and Reich, J. (eds), *The Treatment of Child Molesters*, New York: SBC-TM.

Abel, G. and Becker, J. (1985) 'Sexual Interest Card Sort', in Salter, A. (ed.) (1988) *Treating Child Sex Offenders and Victims – a Practical Guide*, Beverly Hills, CA: Sage.

Abel, G. and Rouleau, J. (1990) 'The Nature and Extent of Sexual Assault', in Marshall, W.L., Laws, D. and Barbaree, H. (eds) *Handbook of Sexual Assualt*, New York: Plenum.

Abel, G., Becker, J., and Cunningham-Rathner, J. (1984) 'Complications, Consent and Cognitions in Sex Between Children and Adults', *International Journal of Law and Psychiatry* 7: 89–103.

Abel, G., Becker, J. and Skinner, L. (1983) 'Behavioral Approaches to Treatment of the Violent Sex Offender', in Roth, L. (ed.) *Clinical Treatment of the Violent Person*, Washington, DC: NIMH Monograph Series.

Abel, G., Becker, J., Cunningham-Rathner, J. and Rouleau, J. (1987) 'Self reported Sex Crimes of 561 Nonincarcerated Paraphiliacs', *Journal of Interpersonal Violence* 2(6): 3–25.

Abel, G., Becker, J., Murphy, W. and Flanagan, B. (1981) 'Identifying Dangerous Child Molesters', in Stuart, R.B. (ed.) *Violent Behaviour*, New York: Brunner/ Mazel.

Abel, G., Mittelman, M., Becker, J., Rathner, J. and Rouleau, J. (1988) 'Predicting Child Molesters' Response to Treatment', *Annals of the New York Academy of Sciences* 528: 223–34.

Abel, G., Becker, J., Cunningham-Rathner, J., Mittelman, M., Rouleau, J., Kaplan, M. and Reich, J. (1984) *The Treatment of Child Molesters*, SBC-TM, 722 West 168th Street, Box 17, New York, N.Y. 10032.

Adamas, C. and Fay, J. (1984) *Nobody Told Me It Was Rape*, Santa Cruz, CA: Network Publications.

Agazarian, Y. and Peters, R. (1981) *The Visible and Invisible Group*, London: Tavistock/Routledge & Kegan Paul.

Aiken, M., Dewar, R., Di Tomaso, N., Hage, J. and Zeitz, G. (1975) *Coordinating Human Services*, San Francisco, CA: Jossey-Bass.

American Humane Association (1978) *National Reporting Study of Child Abuse and Neglect*, Denver, CO: AHA.

American Psychiatric Association (1987) *DSM-111R*, American Psychiatric Association.

Andrews, D., Zinger I., and Hodge, R. (1990) 'Does Correctional Treatment Work?', *Criminology* 28(3).

Araji, S. and Finkelhor, D. (1986) 'Abusers: A Review of the Research', in Finkelhor, D. and associates (eds) *A Sourcebook on Child Sexual Abuse*, Newbury Park, CA: Sage.

Armstrong, L. (1978) *Kiss Daddy Goodnight*, New York: Pocket Books.

Awad, S. and Saunders, E. (1991) 'Male Adolescent Sexual Assaulters: Clinical Observations', *Journal of Interpersonal Violence* 6(4): 446–60.

Badgley, R. (1984) *Sexual Offences Against Children*, Ottawa: Canadian Government Publishing Centre.

Bagley, C. (1992) 'Characteristics of 60 Children and Adolescents with a History of Sexual Assault Against Others: Evidence from a Comparative Study', *Journal of Forensic Psychiatry* 3(2).

Baker, A. and Duncan, S. (1985) 'Child Sexual Abuse: A Study of Prevalence in Great Britain', *Child Abuse and Neglect* 9: 457–67.

Barbaree, H.E. and Marshall, W.L. (1988) 'Deviant Sexual Arousal, Offence History and Demographic Variables as Predictions of Reoffence among Child Molesters', *Behavioural Sciences and the Law* 6: 267–80.

Barbaree, H.E. and Marshall, W.L. (1989) 'Erectile Responses among Heterosexual Child Molesters, Father–Daughter Incest Offenders, and Matched Non-offenders; Five Distinct Age Preference Profiles', *Canadian Journal of Behavioural Sciences* 21: 70–82.

Barbaree, H.E., Marshall, W.L., Yates, E.P. and Lightfoot, L.O. (1983) 'Alcohol Intoxication and Deviant Sexual Arousal in Male Social Drinkers', *Behaviour Research and Therapy* 21: 365–73.

Barbaree, H.E., Marshall, W.L. and Connor, J. (1988) 'The Social Problem Solving of Child Molesters', unpublished manuscript, Queen's University, Kingston, Ontario, Canada.

Barker, M. and Morgan, R. (1993) *Sex Offenders: A Framework for the Evaluation of Community-based Treatment*, London: Home Office.

Barnett, S., Corder, F. and Jehu, D. (1989) 'Group Treatment for Women Sex Offenders' *Practice* 3: 148–59.

Beck, A., Rush, J., Hollon, S. and Shaw, B. (1979) *Cognitive Therapy of Depression*, New York: Guilford Press.

Becker, J.V. and Kaplan, M. (1988) 'The Assessment of Adolescent Sex Offenders', *Advances in Behavioural Assessment of Children and Families* 4: 97–118.

Becker, J.V. and Stein, R.M. (1991) 'Is Sexual Erotica Associated with Sexual Deviance in Adolescent Males?', *International Journal of Law and Psychiatry* 14: 85–95.

Becker, J.V., Kaplan, M. and Kavoussi, R. (1988) 'Measuring the Effectiveness of Treatment for the Aggressive Adolescent Sex Offender', *Annals of the New York Academy of Sciences* 528: 215–22.

Becker, J., Hunter, J., Stein, R. and Kaplan, M. (1989) 'Factors Associated with Erection in Adolescent Sex Offenders', *Journal of Psychopathology and Behavioural Assessment* 11: 4.

Beckett, R. (1993) personal correspondence.

Beckett, R.C., Beech, A., Fisher, D. and Fordham, A.S. (1994) *Community-based*

Treatment for Sex Offenders: An Evaluation of Seven Treatment Programmes, London: Home Office.

Beckett, R., Leck., C., O'Callaghan, D. and Print, B. (in preparation) 'Evaluation of the Effectiveness of Treatment of Adolescent Sex Offenders Referred to the Greater Manchester Adolescent Sex Offender Programme'.

Beckett, R., Leck., C., O'Callaghan, D. and Print, B. (in preparation) 'A Comparative Study of Adolescent Sex Offenders and Non-sexual Offenders in the UK'.

Behroozi, C.S. (1992) 'Groupwork with Involuntary Clients: Remotivating Strategies', *Groupwork* 5(2): 31–41.

Belfer, P.L. and Levendusky, P. (1985) 'Long-term Behavioral Group Psychotherapy – An Integrative Model', in Upper, D. and Ross, S. (eds) *Handbook of Behavioural Group Therapy*, New York: Plenum Press.

Benoit, J.L. and Kennedy, W.A. (1992) 'The Abuse History of Male Adolescent Sex Offenders', *Journal of Interpersonal Violence* 7 (4).

Bentovim, A. (1988) 'Understanding the Phenomenon of Sexual Abuse – A Family Systems View of Causation', in Bentovim, A., Elton, A., Hildebrand, J., Tranter, M. and Vizard, E. (eds) *Child Sexual Abuse Within the Family: Assessment and Treatment. The Work of the Great Ormond Street Sexual Abuse Team*, Bristol: J. Wright.

Berne, E. (1975) *What Do You Say After You Say Hello?*, London: Corgi.

Bion, W.R. (1943) 'Intra-group Tensions in Therapy', *Lancet* 27 November.

Braye, S. (1978) 'Anxiety and Defence in Social Work', unpublished thesis, Exeter University.

Briere, J. and Runtz, M. (1989) 'University Males Sexual Interest in Children: Predicting Potential Indices of "Paedophilia" in a Nonforensic Sample', *Child Abuse and Neglect* 13: 65–75.

Briggs, D. (1979) 'Penile Plethysmographic Measurement of Sexual Arousal in Male Sex Offenders: Effects of Instruction and Varying Stimulus Modality upon Plethysmographic and related Physiological Measures', unpublished M.Sc. thesis, University of Leicester.

Briggs, D. (1992) personal communication.

Brown, A. (1979) *Groupwork*, London: Heinemann.

Butler-Sloss, E. (1988) *The Report of the Inquiry Into Child Abuse in Cleveland, 1987*, London: HMSO, Cmnd 412.

Clyde, (1992) *The Report of the Inquiry into the Removal of Children from Orkney in February 1991*, Edinburgh: HMSO.

Cooke, D., Baldwin, P. and Howison, J. (1990) *Psychology in Prisons*, London: Routledge.

Coons, P.M. and Milstein, V. (1986) 'Psychosexual Disturbances in Multiple Personality: Characteristics, Aetiology and Treatment', *Journal of Clinical Psychiatry* 47(3): 106–10.

Cormier, B. (1988) *The Management and Treatment of Sex Offenders, Report of the Working Group*, Correctional Service of Canada.

Cowburn, M. (1991) 'Sex Offenders in Prison: A Study of Structured Interventions Designed to Change Offending Behaviour', unpublished M. Phil. thesis, University of Nottingham.

Cowburn, M. and Wilson, C. (1992) *Changing Men – A Practice Guide to Working with Adult Male Sex Offenders*, Nottinghamshire Probation Service.

Cranwell-Ward, J.(1987) *Managing Stress*, Aldershot: Gower.

Cross, T. (1991) 'Cross Cultural Competence in Child Protection Work', paper given at 'Excellence in Training' conference, Cornell, July.

Cummings, C., Gordon, J. and Marlatt, G.A. (1980) 'Relapse: Prevention and Prediction', in Miller, W.R. (ed.) *The Addictive Behaviours*, Oxford: Pergamon.

Cunningham, C. and MacFarlane, K. (1991) *When Children Molest Children – Group Treatment Strategies for Young Sexual Abusers*, Orwell, VT: Safer Society Press.

Dacey, R. and Butwell, M. (1991) personal communication.

Darke, J. (1990) 'Sexual Assault; Achieving Power through Humiliation', in Marshall, W., Laws, D., Barbaree, H. (eds) *Handbook of Sexual Assault*, New York: Plenum.

Davies, G.E. and Leitenberg, H. (1987) 'Adolescent Sex Offenders', *Psychological Bulletin* 101: 417–27.

Davis, M.H. (1980) 'A Multi-dimensional Approach to Individual Differences in Empathy', *J.S.A.S. Catalog of Selected Documents in Psychology* 10: 85.

Department of Health (1988) *Protecting Children: A Guide for Social Workers Undertaking a Comprehensive Assessment*, London: HMSO.

Department of Health (1991a) *The Children Act, 1989*, London: HMSO.

Department of Health (1991b) *Working Together under the Children Act 1989*, London: HMSO.

Department of Health (1992) *Strategic Statement on Working with Sex Offenders*, London: HMSO.

Dietz, C.A. and Craft, J.L. (1980) 'Family Dynamics of Incest: A New Perspective', *Social Casework*, 61: 602–9.

Dietz, P.E. (1978) 'Social Factors in Rapist Behaviour', in Rada, R.T. (ed.) *Clinical Aspects of the Rapist*, New York: Grune and Stratton.

Dube, R. and Herbert, M. (1988) 'Sexual Abuse of Children Under 12 Years of Age: A Review of 511 Cases', *Child Abuse and Neglect* 12: 321–30.

Eldridge, H. (1991) *The Sentencing of Sex Offenders, Report of an Interdisciplinary Conference*, London: Suzy Lamplugh Trust.

Elliott, M. (ed.) (1993) *The Ultimate Taboo*, London: Longman.

Elton, A. (1988) 'Assessment of Families for Treatment', in Bentovim, A., Elton, A., Hildebrand, J., Tranter, M. and Vizard, E. (eds) *Child Sexual Abuse Within the Family: Assessment and Treatment. The Work of the Great Ormond Street Sexual Abuse Team*, Bristol: J. Wright.

Erooga, M. (1983) 'Theories and Methods in the Field of Non-accidental Injury to Children: A Study of Some Current Theories and Methods of Intervention and their Application in Different Fieldwork Settings', unpublished MA thesis, University of Manchester.

Erooga, M., Clark, P. and Bentley, M. (1990) 'Protection, Control and Treatment: Groupwork with Child Sexual Abuse Perpetrators', *Groupwork* 3(2): 172–90.

Everson, M., Hunter, W., Runyon, D., Edelson, G. and Coulter, J. (1989) 'Maternal Support Following Disclosure of Incest', *American Journal of Orthopsychiatry* 59(2): 197–207.

Fagan, J. and Wexler, S. (1988) 'Explanations of Sexual Assault Among Violent Delinquents', *Journal of Adolescent Research* 3: 363–85.

Faller, K.C. (1990) *Understanding Child Sexual Maltreatment*, Beverly Hills, CA: Sage.

Farrel, K.J. and O'Brien, B. (eds) (1988) *Sexual Offences by Youths in Michigan: Data, Implications, and Policy Recommendations*, Detroit, MI: Safer Society Resources of Detroit Michigan, Michigan Adolescent Sexual Abuser Project.

Fehrenbach, P. (1983) 'Adolescent Sex Offenders', *Audio Digest of Psychiatry* 12.

Fehrenbach, P., Smith, W., Monastersky, C. and Deisher, R. (1986) 'Adolescent Sex Offenders: Offender and Offence Characteristics', *American Journal of Orthopsychiatry* 56: 225–33.

Fineman, S. (1985) *Social Work Stress and Intervention*, Aldershot: Gower.

Finkelhor, D. (1979) *Sexually Victimised Children*, New York: Free Press.

Finkelhor, D. (1984) *Child Sexual Abuse: New Theory and Research*, New York: Free Press.

Finkelhor, D. and Lewis, I.S. (1988) 'An Epidemiologic Approach to the Study of Child Molestation', in Prentky, R.A. and Quinsey, V. (eds) *Human Sexual Aggression: Current Perspectives*, (vol. 528), New York: New York Academy of Sciences.

Finkelhor, D. and Russell, D. (1984) 'Women as Perpetrators', in Finkelhor, D. (ed.) *Child Sexual Abuse: New Theory and Research*, New York: Free Press.

Forward, S. and Buck, C. (1978) *Betrayal of Innocence: Incest and its Devastation*, London: Penguin.

Freud, S. (1948) *Three Contributions to the Theory of Sex*, 4th edn, New York: Mental Disease Monographs.

Freund, K. (1987) 'Erotic Preference in Paedophiles', *Behaviour Research and Therapy* 5: 339–48.

Friedman, S. and Harrison, G. (1984) 'Sexual Histories, Attitudes and Behaviour of Schizophrenic and "Normal" Women', *Archives of Sexual Behaviour* 13(6): 555–67.

Fritz, G.S., Stoll, K. and Wagner, N. (1981) 'A Comparison of Males and Females who were Molested as Children', *Journal of Sex and Marital Therapy* 7: 54–9.

Fromuth, M. and Burkhart, B. (1987) 'Childhood Sexual Victimisation Among College Men: Definitional and Methodological Issues', *Violence and Victims* 2(4): 241–53.

Fromuth, M.E., Jones, C.W. and Burkhart, B.R. (1991) 'Hidden Child Molestation: An Investigation of Perpetrators in a Non-clinical Sample', *Journal of Interpersonal Violence* 6(3): 376–84.

Furby, L., Weinrott, M.R. and Blackshaw, L. (1989) 'Sex Offender Recidivism: A Review', *Psychological Bulletin* 105: 3–30.

Furniss, T. (1987) 'Organising a Therapeutic Approach to Intrafamilial Child Sexual Abuse', *American Journal of Adolescence* 7.

Garlick, Y. (1991) 'Intimacy Failure, Loneliness and the Attribution of Blame in Sexual Offending', paper presented at UK Prison Service Psychology Conference.

George, W. and Marlatt, G. (1989) 'Introduction to Relapse Prevention with Sexual Offenders', in Laws, D.R. (ed.) *Relapse Prevention with Sexual Offenders*, New York: Guilford Press.

Gibbens, T.C.N., Soothill, K.L. and Way, C.K. (1978) 'Sibling and Parent Incest Offenders', *British Journal of Criminology* 18: 40–52.

Gibbens, T.C.N., Soothill, K.L. and Way, C.K. (1981) 'Sex Offences Against Young Girls: A Long-term Record Study', *Psychological Medicine* 11: 351–7.

Glaser, D. (1991) 'Treatment Issues in Child Sexual Abuse', *British Journal of Psychiatry* 159: 769–82.

Glaser, D. and Frosh, S. (1988) *Child Sexual Abuse*, Basingstoke: BASW/Macmillan.

Goldstein, A.P. and Keller, H., (1987) *Aggressive Behaviour: Assessment and Treatment*, New York: Pergamon.

Gomes-Schwartz, B., Horowitz, J.M. and Caldarelli, A.P. (1990) *Child Sexual Abuse: The Initial Effects*, Beverly Hills, CA: Sage.

Goodchilds, J.D. and Zellman, G.L. (1984) 'Sexual Signalling and Sexual Aggression in Adolescent Relationships', in Malamuth, N.M. and Donnerstein, E. (eds) *Pornography and Sexual Aggression*, Orlando, FL: Academic Press.

Goodman, R.E. (1987) 'Genetic and Hormonal Factors in Human Sexuality: Evolutionary and Developmental Perspectives', in Wilson, G.D. (ed.) *Variant Sexuality: Research and Theory*, Baltimore, MD: Johns Hopkins University Press.

Goring, S. and Ward, R. (1990) 'Groupwork With Sexual Offenders – The Legal Problems', *Journal of Social Welfare* (3): 193–203.

Groth, A.N. (1979) *Men who rape: The psychology of the offender*, New York: Plenum.

Groth, A.N., Longo, R.E. and McFadin, J.B. (1982) 'Undetected Recidivism in Rapists and Child Molesters', *Crime and Delinquency* 28: 450–8.

Grubin, D. and Gunn, J. (1990) *The Imprisoned Rapist and Rape*, London: Institute of Psychiatry.

Hallett, C. and Birchall, E. (1992) *Coordination in Child Protection*, London: HMSO.

Havgaard, J.J. and Tilley, C. (1988) 'Characteristics Predicting Children's Responses to Sexual Encounters with other Children', *Child Abuse and Neglect*, 12.

Health Education Authority (1988) *Stress in the Public Sector*, London: HEA.

Herman, J.L. (1981) *'Father–Daughter Incest'*, Cambridge, MA: Harvard University Press.

Hollin, C.R. and Trower, P. (eds) (1986) *Handbook of Social Skills Training*, vols 1 and 2, Oxford: Pergamon.

Home Office (1988) *British Crime Survey*, London: HMSO.

Home Office (1989) *Report of the Advisory Group on Video-recorded Evidence*, London: HMSO.

Home Office (1990a) 'Cautioning Offenders', Circular 59/90, London: HMSO.

Home Office (1990b) *Criminal Statistics*, London: HMSO.

Home Office (1991) *The Work of the Probation Service with Sex Offenders – Report of a Thematic Inspection*, London: HMSO.

Home Office Probation Service Division (1992) *The Effective Management of Sex Offenders: Report of the Tripartite Seminar 1991*, London: HMSO.

Hooper, C. (1992) *Mothers Surviving Sexual Abuse*, London: Routledge.

Howells, K. (1979) 'Some Meanings of Children for Paedophiles', in Cook, M. and Wilson, F. (eds) *Love and Attraction*, Oxford: Pergamon.

Hunter, J.A. (1991) 'A Comparison of the Psychological Maladjustment of Adult Males and Females Sexually Molested as Children', *Journal of Interpersonal Violence* 6(2): 205–17.

Jesness, D.F. (1962) *The Jesness Inventory*, Palo Alto, CA: Consulting Psychologists Press.

Jones, D. (1993) *Report of the Michael Sieff Conference*, The Michael Sieff Foundation.

Kahn, T.J. and Chambers, H. (1991) 'Assessing Reoffence Risk with Juvenile Sexual Offenders', *Child Welfare* LXX(3).

Kahn, T.J. and Lafond, M.A. (1988) 'Treatment of the Adolescent Sex Offender', *Child and Adolescent Social Work Journal* 5.

Kaplan, M.S. (1985) 'The Impact of Parolees' Perceptions of Confidentiality on the

Reporting of their Urges to Interact Sexually with Children', unpublished doctoral dissertation, New York University.

Kaplan, M., Becker, J. and Cunningham-Rathner, J. (1988) 'Characteristics of Parents of Adolescent Incest Perpetrators: Preliminary Findings', *Journal of Family Violence* 3(3) 183–91.

Kaplan, M.S., Becker, J.V. and Tenke, C.E. (1991) 'Influence of Abuse History on Male Adolescent Self-reported Comfort with Interviewer Gender', *Journal of Interpersonal Violence* 6(1): 3–11.

Kelley, S. (1990) 'Responsibility and Management Strategies in Child Sexual Abuse: A Comparison of Child Protective Workers, Nurses and Police Officers', *Child Welfare* 69(1).

Kelly, L. (1991) *Surviving Sexual Violence*, Cambridge: Polity Press.

Kelly, L., Regan, L. and Burton, S. (1991) *An Exploratory Study of the Prevalence of Sexual Abuse in a Sample of 16–21 Year Olds*, London: CSAU, North London Polytechnic.

Kennedy, M. (1989) 'The Abuse of Deaf Children', *Child Abuse Review*, Spring: 3–7.

Kerr, L. (1991) 'Probation Practice with Sex Offenders: An Analysis of the Stresses On and the Coping Strategies Used by Probation Officers', unpublished MA thesis, University of Sheffield.

Knight, R.A., Carter, D.L., and Prentky, R.A. (1989) 'A System for the Classification of Child Molesters. Reliability and Application, *Journal of Interpersonal Violence* 4: 3–23.

Knight, R.K. (1988) 'A Taxonomic Analysis of Child Molesters', in Prentky, R.A. and Quinsey, V. (eds) *Human Sexual Aggression: Current Perspectives*, New York: New York Academy of Sciences.

Knopp, F.H. (1988) *Remedial Intervention in Adolescent Sex Offences: Nine Program Descriptions*, Syracuse, NY: Safer Society Press.

Knopp, F.H., Freeman Longo, R. and Stevenson, W.F. (1992) *Nationwide Survey of Juvenile and Adult Sex Offender Treatment Program and Models*, Orwell, VT: Safer Society Program Publications.

Korda, L. and Pancrazio, J. (1989) 'Limiting Negative Outcome in Group Practice', *The Journal for Specialists in Groupwork* 14(2): 112–20.

Lane, S. (1986) 'Potential Emotional Hazards of Working with Sex Offenders', *Interchange*, January, Denver, CO: Kempe Center.

Lane, S. and Zamora, P. (1978) Syllabus Materials from Inservice Training on Adolescent Sex Offenders; Closed Adolescent Treatment Center, Denver, CO: Division of Youth Services.

Langevin, R., Handy, L., Day, D. and Russon, A. (1985) 'Are Incestuous Fathers Paedophilic, Aggressive and Alcoholic?', in Langevin, R. (ed.) *Erotic Preference, Gender Identity and Aggression*, Hillsdale, NJ: Erlbaum.

Lankester, D. and Meyer, B. (1986) 'Relationship of Family Structure to Sex Offence Behaviour', paper presented at First National Conference on Juvenile Sexual Offending, Minneapolis, MN.

Lanyon, R.I., Dannenbaum, S.E. and Brown, R.A.R. (1991) 'Detection of Deliberate denial in Child Abusers', *Journal of Interpersonal Violence* 6(3): 301–9.

Laws, D.R. (ed.) (1989) *Relapse Prevention with Sexual Offenders*, New York: Guilford Press.

Laws, D.R. and Marshall, W.L. (1990) 'A Conditioning Theory of the Etiology and Maintenance of Deviant Sexual Preference and Behaviour', in Marshall,

W.L., Laws, D.R. and Barbaree, H.E. (eds) *Handbook of Sexual Assault*, New York: Plenum.

Laws, D.R. and Marshall, W.L. (1991) 'Masturbatory Reconditioning with Sexual Deviates: An Evaluative Review', *Advances in Behavioural Research and Therapy* 13: 13–25.

Liberman, R.P., King, L.W., De Ris, W.J. and McCann, M.J. (1975) *Personal Effectiveness Training: Guiding People to Assert their Feelings and Improve their Social Skills*, Champaign, IL: Research Press.

Lipsey, M. (1990) 'Juvenile Delinquency Treatment', in *Meta Analysis for Exploration: A Casebook*, Russell Sage Foundation.

McCarthy, L. (1981) 'Investigation of Incest: Opportunity to Motivate Families to Seek Help', *Child Welfare* 60: 679–89.

McColl, A. and Hargreaves, R. (1992) 'Explaining Sex Offending in Court Reports', *Probation Journal* 40(1).

McCraw, R.K. and Pegg-McNab, J. (1989) 'Rorschach Comparisons of Male Juvenile Sex Offenders and Non-sex Offenders', *Journal of Personality Assessment* 53(3).

McFall, R.M. (1990) 'The Enhancement of Social Skills: An Information Processing Analysis', in Marshall, W.L., Laws, D.R. and Barbaree, H.E. (eds) *Handbook of Sexual Assault*, New York: Plenum.

McGrath, R. (1990) 'Assessment of Sexual Aggressors: Practical Clinical Interviewing Strategies, *Journal of Interpersonal Violence* 5: 507–19.

McGrath, R.J. (1991) 'Sex Offender Risk Assessment and Dispositional Planning: A Review of Empirical and Clinical Findings', *International Journal of Offender Therapy Comparative Criminology* 35(4): 328–50.

McIvor, G. (1990) *Solutions for Serious or Persistent Offenders; A Review of the Literature*, University of Stirling Social Work Research Centre.

Malamuth, N.M. (1981) 'Rape Proclivity among Males', *Journal of Social Issues* 37: 138–57.

Maletzky, B.M. (1990) *Treating the Sexual Offender*, Beverly Hills, CA: Sage.

Manning, H. (1992) *Adolescent Sex Offender Treatment Programme*, Victoria, Australia: Young Offender Health Services.

Margolin, L. (1993) 'In their Parents' Absence: Sexual Abuse in Child Care', *Violence Update 3(9)*.

Marlatt, G.A. and Gordon, J.R. (1985) (eds) *Relapse Prevention. Maintenance Strategies in the Treatment of Addictive Behaviors*, New York: Guilford Press.

Marshall, W.L. and Barbaree, H.E. (1990a) 'Outcome of Cognitive-behavioural Treatment', in Marshall, W.L., Laws, D.R. and Barbaree, H.E. (eds) *Handbook of Sexual Assault*, New York: Plenum.

Marshall, W. L. and Barbaree, H.E. (1990b) 'Present State and Future Direction', in Marshall, W.L., Laws, D.R. and Barbaree, H.E. (eds) *Handbook of Sexual Assault*, New York: Plenum.

Marshall, W.L. and Eccles, A. (1991) 'Issues in Clinical Practice with Sex Offenders', *Journal of Interpersonal Violence* 6: 68–93.

Marshall, W.L., Barbaree, H.E. and Christopher, D. (1986) 'Sexual Offenders against Female Children: Preferences for Age of Victim and Type of Behaviour', *Canadian Journal of Behavioural Science* 18: 424–39.

Marshall, W.L., Barbaree, H.E. and Eccles, A. (1991) 'Early Onset and Deviant Sexuality in Child Molesters', *Journal of Interpersonal Violence* 6(3): 323–36.

Marshall, W. L., Bates, L. and Rhule, M. (1984) 'Hostility in Sex Offenders', unpublished manuscript, Queen's University, Kingston, Ontario, Canada.

Marshall, W.L., Hudson, S.M. and Ward, T. (in press) 'Sexual Deviance', in Wilson, P.D. (ed.) *Principles and Practice of Relapse Prevention*, New York: Guilford Press.

Marshall, W., Laws, D. and Barbaree, H.E. (eds) (1990) *Handbook of Sexual Assault*, New York: Plenum.

Marshall, W.L., Ward, T., Jones, R., Johnston, P. and Barbaree, H.E. (1991) 'An Optimistic Evaluation of Treatment Outcome with Sex Offenders', *Violence Update* 1(7): 1, 8, 10–11.

Masson H. and Erooga, M. (1989) 'Take A Break', *Community Care*, 7 December: 792.

Mathews, R., Mathews, J.K. and Speltz, K. (1989) *Female Sexual Offenders: An Exploratory Study*, Orwell, VT: Safer Society Press.

Mattinson, J. and Sinclair, I. (1979) *Mate and Stalemate*, London: IMS/Blackwell.

Mehrabian, A. and Epstein N. (1972) 'A Measure of Emotional Empathy', *Journal of Personality* 40: 525–9.

Menzies, I. (1970) 'A Case Study in the Functioning of Social Systems as a Defence Against Anxiety', *Social Relations* 13(2).

Miller, W. (1983) 'Motivational Interviewing with Problem Drinkers', *Behavioural Psychotherapy* 11: 147–72.

Morrison, T. (1990) 'The Emotional Effects of Child Protection Work on the Worker' *Practice* 4(4).

Morrison, T. (1992) Managing Sex Offenders: The Challenge for Managers, *Probation Journal* 39(3).

Morrison, T. (1993) personal communication.

Muehlenard, C.L. and Linton, M.A. (1987) 'Date Rape and Sexual Aggression in Dating Situations: Incidence and Risk Factors', *Journal of Counselling Psychology* 34: 186–96.

Murphy, W. D., Haynes, M.R., Stalgaitis, S.J. and Flanagan, B. (1986) 'Differential Sexual Responding amongst Four Groups of Sexual Offenders against Children', *Journal of Psychopathology and Behavioural Assessment* 8: 339–53.

Murrey, G.J., Briggs, D. and Davis, C. (1992) 'Psychopathic Disordered, Mentally Ill and Mentally Handicapped Sex Offenders: A Comparative Study, *Medicine, Science and the Law* 32(4): 331–6.

Nash, C.L. and West, D.J. (1985) 'Sexual Molestation of Young Girls: A Retrospective Study', in West, D.J. (ed.) *Sexual Victimisation*, Aldershot: Gower.

National Adolescent Perpetrator Network (NAPN) (1988) 'Preliminary Report from the National Task Force on Juvenile Sexual Offending', *Juvenile and Family Court Journal* 39(2).

National Centre on Child Abuse and Neglect (NCCAN) (1981) *Study of National Incidence and Prevalence of Child Abuse and Neglect*, Washington, DC: US Department of Health and Human Services.

National Children's Homes (1992) *Report of the Committee of Enquiry into Children and Young People who Sexually Abuse Other Children*, London: NCH.

Nelson, S. (1982) *Incest – Fact and Myth*, Edinburgh: Stramullion.

Nichols, H.R. and Molinder, I. (1984) *Multiphasic Sex Inventory Manual*, Tacoma, WA: Authors.

North West Treatment Associates (1988) in Salter, A. *Treating Child Sex Offenders and Victims – A Practical Guide*, Beverly Hills, CA: Sage.

Northern Ireland Research Team (1991) *Child Sexual Abuse in Northern Ireland*, Belfast: Greystone.

Novaco, R.W. (1979) 'The Cognitive Regulation of Anger and Stress' in Kendall, P.C. and Hollon, S.D. (eds) *Cognitive-behavioural Interventions; Theory, Research and Procedures*, London: Academic Press.

O'Brien, M. (1991) 'Taking Sibling Incest Seriously', in Quinn-Patton, M. (ed.) *Family Sexual Abuse: Frontline Research and Evaluation*, Beverly Hills, CA: Sage.

O'Connell, M., Leberg, E. and Donaldson, C. (1990) *Working with Sex Offenders: Guidelines for Therapist Selection*, Beverly Hills, CA: Sage.

Olafson, E., Corwin, D. and Summit, R. (1993) 'Modern History of Child Sexual Abuse Awareness: Cycles of Discovery and Suppression', *Child Abuse and Neglect* 17: 7–24.

Overholsen, J.C. and Beck, S. (1986) 'Multimethod Assessment of Rapists, Child Molesters and Three Control Groups on Behavioural and Psychological Measures', *Journal of Consulting and Clinical Psychology* 54: 682–7.

Panton, J.H. (1978) 'Personality Differences Appearing Between Rapists of Adults, Rapists of Children and Non-violent Sexual Molesters of Children', *Research Communications in Psychology, Psychiatry and Behaviour* 3(4): 385–93.

Parker, H. (1984) '*Intrafamilial Sexual Child Abuse. A Study of the Abusive Father*', Doctoral Dissertation, University of Utah, Dissertation Abstracts International 45,123757A

Parker, H. and Parker, S. (1986) 'Father–Daughter Sexual Abuse. An Emerging Perspective', *American Journal of Orthopsychiatry* 56: 531–49.

Peake, A. (1989a) *Outline for Monitoring Young Children in Schools*, London: Children's Society.

Peake, A. (1989b) *Outline for Monitoring Children in Secondary Schools*, London: Children's Society.

Petras (1973) *Sexuality and Society*

Petty, G.M. and Dawson, B. (1989) 'Sexual Aggression in Normal Men: Incidence, Beliefs and Personality Characteristics', *Personality and Individual Differences* 10(3): 355–62.

Phillpotts, G.J.O. and Lancucki, L.B. (1979) *Previous Convictions, Sentence and Reconviction*, London: HMSO.

Pierce, L.H. and Pierce, R.L. (1990) 'Adolescent/Sibling Incest Perpetrators', in Horton, L., Johnson, B., Roundy, L. and Williams, D. (eds) *The Incest Perpetrator: A Family Member No One Wants To Treat*, Beverly Hills, CA: Sage.

Pines, A.M., Aronson, E. and Kafry, D. (1981) *Burnout: From Tedium to Growth*, New York: Free Press.

Pithers, W. (1990) 'Relapse Prevention with Sexual Aggressors', in Marshall, W., Laws, D. and Barbaree, H. (eds) *Handbook of Sexual Assault*, New York: Plenum.

Pithers. W. and Cumming, G. (1989) 'Can Relapses be Prevented? Initial Outcome Data from the Vermont Treatment Programme for Sexual Aggression', in Laws, D.R. (ed.) *Relapse Prevention with Sex Offenders*, New York, Guilford Press.

Pithers, W.D., Kashima, K., Cumming, G.F., Beal, L.S. and Buell, M. (1988) 'Relapse Prevention of Sexual Aggression', in Prentky, R. and Quinsey, V. (eds) *Human Sexual Aggression Current Perspectives*, New York: New York Academy of Sciences.

Preston-Shoot, M. and Braye, S. (1991) 'Managing the Personal Experience of Work' *Practice* 5(1).

Probation Service Division/ACOP (1992) 'Supervision of Sex Offenders', *ACOP* 52.

Prochaska, J. and Di Clemente, C. (1982) 'Transtheoretical Therapy: Toward a more Integrative Model of Change', *Psychotherapy: Theory, Research and Practice* 19(3).

Quinsey, V.L. and Earls, C.M. (1990) 'The Modification of Sexual Preferences', in Marshall, W.L., Laws, D.R. and Barbaree, H.E. (eds) *Handbook of Sexual Assault*, New York: Plenum.

Quinsey, V.L., Chaplin, T.C. and Carrigan, W.F. (1979) 'Sexual Preferences amongst Incestuous and Nonincestuous Child Molesters', *Behaviour Therapy* 10: 562–5.

Quinsey, V.L., Chaplin, T.C. and Varney, G. (1981) 'A Comparison of Rapists' and Non-sex Offenders' Sexual Preferences for Mutually Consenting Sex, Rape and Physical Abuse of Women', *Behavioural Assessment* 3: 127–35.

Rada, R.T. (1978) *Clinical Aspects of the Rapist*, New York: Grune and Stratton.

Rapaport, K. and Burkhart, B.R. (1984) 'Personality and Attitudinal Characteristics of Sexually Coercive College Males', *Journal of Abnormal Psychology* 93: 216–21.

Roberts, C. (1991) *What Works: Using Social Work Methods to Reduce Reoffending in Serious and Persistent Offenders*, Oxford: Applied Social Studies, University of Oxford.

Rosenthal, J.A., Motz, J.K., Edmonson, D.A. and Groze, V. (1991) 'A Descriptive Study of Abuse and Neglect in Out of Home Placement', *Child Abuse and Neglect* 13: 249–60.

Ross, J.E. (1990) *Correctional Sex Offender Treatment Program Guide-Lines*, South Carolina, Jonathan E. Ross, M.A. Inc.

Russell, D. (1983) 'The Incidence and Prevalence of Intrafamilial and Extra Familial Sexual Abuse of Female Children', *Child Abuse and Neglect* 7: 133–46.

Russell, D. (1984) *The Secret Trauma: Incest in the Lives of Girls and Women*, New York: Basic Books.

Ryan, G. and Lane, S. (eds) (1991) *Juvenile Sexual Offending – Causes, Consequences and Corrections*, Lexington, MA: Lexington Books.

Ryan, G., Lane, S.R., Davis, J.M. and Isaac, C.B. (1987) 'Juvenile Sex Offenders: Development and Correction', *Child Abuse and Neglect* 2: 385–95.

Salter, A. (1988) *Treating Child Sex Offenders and Victims – A Practical Guide*, Beverly Hills, CA: Sage.

Salter, A. (1992) *NOTA Conference Proceedings*, Dundee.

Sarafino, E.P. (1979) 'An Estimate of Nationwide Incidence of Sexual Offences Against Children', *Child Welfare* 587(2): 127–34.

Saunders, D.G. (1991) 'Procedures for Adjusting Self-reports of Violence for Social Desirability Bias', *Journal of Interpersonal Violence* 6(3): 336–44.

Saunders, E.B. and Awad, G.A. (1988) 'Assessment, Management and Treatment Planning for Male Adolescent Sexual Offenders', *American Journal of Orthopsychiatry* 58(4).

Sawyer, J. (1966) 'Measurement and Prediction: Clinical and Statistical', *Psychological Bulletin* 66: 178–200.

Sefarbi, R. (1990) 'Admitters and Deniers Among Adolescent Sex Offenders and their Families', *American Journal of Orthopsychiatry* 60(3).

Segal, Z.V. and Marshall, W.L. (1985) 'Self Report and Behavioural Assertion in Five Groups of Sexual Offenders', *Behaviour Therapy and Experimental Psychiatry* 16(3): 223–9.

Sgroi, S. (1982) *Handbook of Clinical Intervention in Child Sexual Abuse*, Lexington, MA: Lexington Books.

Sgroi, S. (ed.) (1989) *Vulnerable Populations*, vol. 1, Lexington, MA: Lexington Books.

Sheath, M. (1990) 'Confrontative Work with Sex Offenders: Legitimised Nonce-bashing?', *Probation Journal* 37(4).

Simon, W.T. and Schouter, P.G.W. (1992) 'Problems in Sexual Preference Testing in Child Sexual Abuse Cases: A Legal and Community Perspective', *Journal of Interpersonal Violence 7(4): 503–16*.

Smets, A.C. and Cebula, C.M. (1987) 'A Group Treatment Program for Adolescent Sex Offenders: Five Steps toward Resolution', *Child Abuse and Neglect* 2: 247–54.

Smith, H. and Israel, E. (1987) 'Sibling Incest: A Study of the Dynamics of 25 Cases', *Child Abuse and Neglect* 2.

Smith, W.R. (1988) 'Delinquency and Abuse Among Juvenile Sexual Offenders', *Journal of Interpersonal Violence* 3(4).

Soothill, K.L. and Gibbens, T.C.N. (1978) 'Recidivism of Sex Offenders: A Reappraisal', *British Journal of Criminology* 18(3): 267–76.

Steen, C. and Monnette, B. (1989) *Treating Adolescent Sex Offenders in the Community*, Springfield, IL: Thomas Books.

Spence, J. and Helmreich, R. (1972) 'The Attitudes Toward Women Scale: An Objective Instrument to Measure Attitudes Toward the Rights and Roles of Women in Contemporary Society', *Psychological Documents* 2: 153.

Sullivan, H. (1953) *The Interpersonal Theory of Psychiatry*, New York: Norton.

Summit, R. (1983) 'The Child Sexual Abuse Accommodation Syndrome', *Child Abuse and Neglect* 7: 177–93.

Thornton, D. (1991) *Treatment of Sexual Offenders in Prison: A Strategy*, Directorate of Inmate Programmes, HM Prison Service, Monograph.

Thornton, D. and Travers, R. (1991) 'A Longitudinal Study of the Criminal Behaviour of Convicted Sexual Offenders', paper presented at Prison Psychologists' Conference, Scarborough.

Through The Maze (1991), distributed by the Albany Video Project, London.

Tuckman, D. (1965) 'Developmental Sequence in Small Groups', *Psychological Bulletin* LXIII: 384–99.

Turk, D. and Salovey, P. (eds) (1988) *Reasoning, Inference, and Judgment in Clinical Psychology*, New York: Free Press.

UN Convention on the Rights of the Child (1989), London: HMSO/UNICEF.

US National Task Force Report on Juvenile Sexual Offending (1988) 'Preliminary Report', *Juvenile and Family Court Journal* 39(2).

Vinogradov, S., Dishotsky, N.I., Doty, A.K. and Tinklenberg, J.R. (1988) 'Patterns of Behaviour in Adolescent Rape', *American Journal of Orthopsychiatry* 58: 179–87.

Wakefield, H. and Underwager, R. (1988) *Accusations of Child Sexual Abuse*, Springfield, IL: Charles C. Thomas.

Wallace, M. (1979) *Black Macho and the Myth of the Superwoman*, London: John Calder.

Watson, D. and Friend, R. (1969) 'Measurement of Social Evaluation Anxiety', *Journal of Consulting and Clinical Psychology* 33(4): 448–57.

Wattam, C. (1993) 'Kids on Film', *Community Care*, 7 October.

Weiner, R. (1989) 'Stress within the Team', *Social Work Today* 20(35): 20–1.

Weinrott, M.R. and Saylor, M. (1991) 'Self-report of Crimes Committed by Sex Offenders', *Journal of Interpersonal Violence* 6(3): 286–300.

Wiehe, V.R. (1990) *Sibling Abuse: Hidden Physical, Emotional and Sexual Trauma*, Lexington, MA: Lexington Books.

Wilson, G. (1978) *The Secrets of Sexual Fantasy,* London: Dent.

Williams. C., Hayes, M., Battersby, G. and Crow, I. (1992) *Acting in Child Protection Cases*, University of Sheffield.

Wolf, S.C. (1984) 'A Multifactor Model of Deviant Sexuality', paper presented at Third International Conference on Victimology, Lisbon.

Woolfe Report (1991), in *The Sentencing of Sex Offenders: Report of an Interdisiplinary Conference*, London: Suzy Lamplugh Trust.

Working Group Sex Offender Treatment Review (1988) *The Management and Treatment of Sex Offenders*, Canada: Ministry of the Solicitor General.

Wyatt, G. (1985) 'The Sexual Abuse of Afro-American and White American Women in Childhood', *Child Abuse and Neglect* 9: 507–19.

Yalom, I. (1975) *The Theory and Practice of Group Psychotherapy* (2nd edn), New York: Basic Books.

Yates, C. (1990) 'A Family Affair: Sexual Offences, Sentencing and Treatment', *Journal of Child Law*, April/July: 70–6.

Yates, E., Barbaree, H.E. and Marshall, W.L. (1984) 'Anger and Deviant Sexual Arousal', *Behaviour Therapy* 15: 287–94.

Index

Abel, G. 1, 6–10 *passim*, 21, 27, 61, 67, 73, 95, 113, 135, 196; cognition scale (with Becker) 71; recidivism data 13, 14, 15; sexual interest card sort (with Becker) 74; surveillance group approach 100
abstinence violation effect 94
abusers 171–2; of boys 57, 74; of boys and girls 12, 13; care-givers 151; child's attachment to 36; convicted, themselves abused sexually as children 7; diagnosed as psychotic 164; differentiating sexual preferences of 73; disclosure by 161; experiences of victimisation 154; extra-familial 57, 73–4, 64, 66, 84, 151; family networks 111; female acting alone 11; fixated 74; of girls 57, 74; identified as victimised 151; intra-familial 57, 66, 73–4, 84; living with victims 159; multiple victims 30; needs for power, acceptance and aggression 156; potential levels in the population 4–6; sexually abused as children 64; stepfathers 155; *see also* adolescent sexual abusers
'abuse-distorted attachments' 36
access to children 23, 66, 92, 151
ACPCs (Area Child Protection Committees) 29, 179, 186
Adamas, C. 147
adolescence: delinquency in 64; early, special emotional or sexual relationships with other children during 70; misrepresentation of

normal peer group behaviour 69; school and employment record 163; sexual experiences 75; *see also* adolescent sexual abusers
adolescent sexual abusers 18, 27, 146–77; abused by males 151; access to victims 151, 152; ages of 149, 150; characteristics of 152–5; child-focused arousal and fantasies developed during 74; cognitive distortions 162; details of sexual fantasies, sexual knowledge and experiences 161; extra-familial 155; female 157; imprisoned 144; intra-familial 151, 152, 154, 155; lack of detection 152; more likely multiple victims 152; offence characteristics 150 151; opportunistic offending 23; personal history of sexual abuse 150; resistance to admitting fantasies 173–4; restricted contact with children 163; sexual violation in institutional care 144; siblings of 172; victim preference 150
adoptive sisters 151
affection 226; bribes of 24; parental, lack of 71
Agazarian, Y. 119–21
age: abusers between ten and nineteen years 149; abusers less than fifteen years 149, 150; age-appropriate partners 65; age of victims 150; Appeal Court sentencing guidelines in cases of incest 225–6; multiple offence categories 9–10; sixteen